The Women of The Rose

The story of mammograms, miracles and a
Texas nonprofit that beat all the odds

Dorothy Gibbons

Designed by Diane Reina

Manufactured in the United States of America

First Printing September, 2015

ISBN: 1515350908

This book chronicles the history of The Rose as seen through my eyes throughout the thirty years that I served as its co-founder and CEO. Some of these stories have been shared in our newsletters, in local newspapers or on television, but others have never been told publicly. These stories are true as remembered by me and from my point of view. Some names and identifying characteristics have been changed to protect the privacy of certain individuals. While a portion of the proceeds from every book sold will benefit The Rose, no funding from The Rose was used in the production of this book.

Dedication

On a sunny spring day, George was driving our newest mobile mammography van from Phoenix to Houston. Our logo and the van's bright pink color could be seen for miles. About twenty miles outside of El Paso, he stopped at a service station. A beat-up pick-up truck pulled up beside him and the driver pushed a dollar bill at him, saying "For The Rose!"

George tried to explain that he was just a driver but the man kept pushing the dollar toward him. In broken English, the man explained that The Rose had taken care of his mother. He would not leave and kept insisting: "For The Rose. They need this."

Finally George took the crumpled bill and sat it on the dashboard.

That dollar bill traveled 800 miles before being placed in my hands.

This book is dedicated to that man's mother and to all the other women of The Rose.

Chapter 1
Orientation
February 16, 2011

I glanced at the clock on the wall; it was 11:35 a.m., and only three more hours until the conference call with the board of directors. I wasn't looking forward to that call, a decision had to be made and it was one I could not make alone. It was a decision that could mean life or death for this organization and was without a doubt the biggest challenge The Rose had ever faced.

After 25 years, I was intimate with the needs of this entity called The Rose and her future was at stake. I had to do what was best for her.

In spite of the current situation, I had to smile to myself, thinking about how I had made the organization a 'she' in my mind. Like most women, she was fickle; the lover who sometimes adored you then totally ignored you. She was a demanding employer, never satisfied, always reminding me that there was still more to do, more people needing help, more lives that would be lost if I didn't give my all and then some. No effort ever met the mark, no amount of hours worked or wishes made would ever be enough.

She was without a doubt the very best thing that had ever come into my life and, if the truth be known, a pretty darn good thing for the 400,000 women we had served, especially the uninsured.

On that morning in 2011, I was in the conference room with seven new employees of The Rose who were completing their day of orientation. The women sitting around the table ranged in age from 22 years old to 58, and they were white, Black, Hispanic, and Asian, as diverse in their personal heritage as in their healthcare experience.

But they shared a common trait; most had never worked in an organization where a single employee had such a direct impact on another person's life. In the months ahead, thousands of women would depend on them knowing how to do their jobs, how to find resources when there were none, how to listen to the real message when a woman said "something doesn't feel right," and how to fit one more appointment into a packed schedule.

They also had no clue about our current struggle or the fact that this might be the last orientation day we would ever hold at The Rose. I quickly pushed that thought from my mind.

"We have a saying around here that you didn't pick The Rose," I said, pausing to look into the eyes of each new employee, "she picked you," I smiled. "For some of you it was because you needed to be here, and for others it is because we needed you."

Two employees exchanged glances, eyebrows raised. The others continued to watch me politely, but it was easy to see the question mark forming in their eyes.

Each month, we set aside a whole morning for orientation, introducing our new employees to the key players, explaining who did what and what our mission was all about. I was always the last speaker for the day. My job was to talk about the history of The Rose, how it began and why our community needed us so badly.

Using the organization chart with its colored-coded squares, I explained how each position related in one way or another to providing medical care to the uninsured. Providing access to care, for any woman, was the heart of our work.

I knew exactly how many people, insured and uninsured, we had served in the past twelve months; the statistics were both impressive and chilling. Of the 33,605 total women and 166 men; 9,496 were uninsured. This was the third year in a row that we had cared for over 9,000 uninsured women. That number was staggering, especially considering that The Rose was among the few remaining 'freestanding' mammography facilities in the nation.

We had two locations in Houston; one was the building we—and the bank—owned that served as our main headquarters. The other was a leased space located more in town. Our mobile mammography vans covered 24 counties in Southeast Texas. The Rose's only focus was breast cancer, we provided mammograms, ultrasounds, biopsies, and physician consults. In fact, our screening and diagnostic services added up to over 60,000 procedures in the past year.

Our patient navigation program ensured that every patient, insured or not, had access to treatment. For the 359 women we had diagnosed during the past year, our ability to move them into timely treatment meant their survival.

"The Rose is not part of a big national organization," I told the new employees. "We don't have the backing of a large medical center to carry us. We don't depend on the government for support. Our annual budget is over $8 million. About $5 million comes from insured women but we have to raise the rest, $3 million each year, from grants and fundraisers to provide services to the uninsured. Every year we start at a zero balance. And whether we succeed or fail is up to us."

Heads nodded.

In front of me on the table sat a black three-ring binder, full of eight by ten photographs, charts, and maps, each held securely in place by clear protector sheets. I ran my fingers over the cover as if I could reach back and touch all the years contained within it and pull out a single memory that would mean something to this group of people.

They would never know what it was like during those early years. They would never wonder if they would get a paycheck that week, or be asked to vacuum floors and clean bathrooms, or have to work at a rickety folding table because a desk hadn't been donated yet. Each of these new folks would have a desk to work from, a phone to use and their own computer, some with two monitors to help with scheduling. Both of our locations were first class, with all the amenities of any modern medical facility.

The black binder was my little time capsule. It sat between me and my new staff, my substitute for a crystal ball. I gazed at it, seeing images from the past and glimpses of the future.

"One thing you need to know is that I'm a feminist." Nervous laughter filled the room. "Now don't get me wrong, I like men, I love my husband and my son and I like the men who work here—well, most of the time," I smiled.

The group laughed.

My tone turned serious. "I believe we have an obligation to be the voice for women, especially for those women who do not have a voice." I paused, wondering if there were any women sitting around the table who still didn't have a voice, in her life or her home.

"Women are smart. They know they need to take care of their bodies, and they would if they could. But too many women, especially those we sponsor, have put everyone else first. They took care of the kids, the family, parents, and they didn't take care of themselves. I bet there isn't a person here who hasn't been without health insurance at some point in her life," heads nodded, "or who hasn't had to watch a family member or friend struggle through some awful disease without insurance and maybe even without getting care.

"Our job is to be a place where women are able to feel safe and where they can keep their dignity. It's hard to ask for help, and we sure aren't going to make it any harder. Let me tell you how The Rose started.

"In the mid-'80s, the oil bust had just about crippled Houston, people were laid off, most had lost their insurance and many were losing their homes, foreclosures were rampant. I worked at Pasadena Bayshore Hospital, which was the tenth largest hospital in Houston, with 500 beds and 1,100 employees. As the public relations director, my job was to market the hospital. Bayshore was a general community hospital, and the biggest thing I could find to market was our birthing center and free baby car seats.

"All that changed in 1983 when Dr. Dixie Melillo came on staff. I finally had SOMETHING to market. Dr. Dixie was a general surgeon and the first female doctor on Bayshore's active medical staff. Pasadena had a reputation for being a tad bit redneck and full of pickup trucks and good ol' boys. I knew that culture well." I smiled at the group, leaning forward and assuming a conspirator's voice. "Look, I raised my son in Pasadena and my family comes from there, so I can say these things!" They all laughed. My son David was seventeen when I met Dixie. I had divorced his dad and moved to Clear Lake years before that, but the work at the hospital kept me tied to that city.

"So, there was Dixie, our new general surgeon. And not only was she a WOMAN, she was a knockout. I always thought she was the most beautiful woman alive. Dixie is tall, and even taller in her high heels—which she always wore. She was so very proper then." I paused at this point in the story and lowered my voice. "She isn't anymore."

The group giggled. Most of the new employees had already met Dixie, these days she lived in scrubs, nice patterned scrubs to match the season of the year, but still scrubs. I couldn't remember the last time I'd seen her in a suit. High heels were a thing of the past. Years of standing, doing surgeries for hours on end, had caused neuropathy in her feet, and now comfortable, open-toed earth shoes were her attire of choice.

Back in the '80s, her suits were gorgeous and she always wore her skirts a little too tight and a little too short. Her necklaces and earrings were perfectly matched, and she never went anywhere without her lipstick, a tube tucked away in the pocket of her lab coat. I would see her coming out of the operating room, her lipstick already freshened, her hair perfect, every strand back in place, looking like she'd stepped out of a fashion magazine.

But the most beautiful thing about Dixie was her passion for breast cancer. After being a resident at UTMB Galveston and seeing hundreds of uninsured women in the late stages of the disease, she was determined to do breast cancer the 'right way.' The first time I ever saw Dixie, she was rounding the corner at Bayshore and moving straight through the crowd that had gathered around the Emergency Room doors. There was no missing her, she stood a full head and shoulders taller than her scrub nurse Peggy walking beside her. Dixie's dark hair was a sharp contrast to her white lab coat and Peggy's blond locks. Her walk was quick, her stride long. Heads turned as she glided past. Dixie's flashing deep-set blue eyes caught folks by surprise with a directness that bored into them.

As the ER doors slowly closed, a crowd of people swarmed around her. She was like a magnet. The nurses quickly surrounded her, charts in hand, while family members stood around the outer edge, anxious lines on their faces starting to dissolve.

"Who's that?" I asked my friend Hazel, the director of medical records.

"Haven't you heard?" Hazel was surprised I hadn't already met this newcomer, but then Hazel had a way of knowing about most anything long before I ever did. "She's the new doctor on staff, from Galveston." Then she emphasized, "A general surgeon."

"A female general surgeon? Wow. How'd they let that happen?" I teased.

"She bought out Dr. Epstein's practice. I understand she's already got the good ol' boys in a bit of a frenzy."

"How so?" I asked.

"Seems she had just finished her surgery in OR and was sitting at that little desk outside in the corridor, working on her post-op notes. One of the guys thought she was a nurse using the space reserved for docs and started making noises. That's when Peggy jumped in, introduced Dixie as DOCTOR Melillo, and told him the doctor would move when the doctor was finished!"

We laughed.

Promoting new physicians was one of my better duties and Dixie hadn't been on staff for very long before I was called to a meeting. As I walked into the administrator's office, I heard her pitch for a new service that no other hospital was offering, at least not in our community.

"You cannot x-ray a woman's breasts with the same machine that's used to x-ray a broken arm," Dixie argued. "You have to have a dedicated mammography unit." She stood in front of the administrator's desk, towering over him, with Joyce, the director of radiology. They were making a pretty convincing case to the administrator.

Women's Health was the latest healthcare marketing rage and Dixie and Joyce pelted him with ideas and facts. "Think of all the great publicity. It's a consumer driven market. It will appeal to every woman."

The administrator was genuinely open to the idea. Of course, he didn't realize that the radiologists had not yet been persuaded of this need. He couldn't have guessed how enraged they would become when they discovered that a general surgeon was actually making suggestions for radiological equipment, and very expensive equipment at that.

"Charging $160 for a mammogram is too much money," Dixie fumed. "Make it a reasonable amount and I'll go out and drum up business for you. I'll give talks to the community. I'll promote it to the hilt, and I promise you I'll get the women in here…in droves!"

"What's reasonable?" the administrator asked.

He shouldn't have said that. One should never ask Dixie what's reasonable, especially when it comes to charges. She wanted it to be $50, he choked on $100, but finally they agreed on $80 per mammogram.

So the deal was struck, the machine ordered, and the marketing plan created. The radiologists balked every step of the way, but soon realized they were starting to look like the bad guys.

No matter how they tried to stop the project, there was no way to halt Dixie's momentum or her growing popularity.

When Bayshore opened the first dedicated breast-imaging center in Pasadena, the publicity was incredible. I soon had Dixie booked out for months with speaking engagements. I produced her slides and carried a big old slide projector and an even bigger screen. I didn't know it then, but I learned that Dixie NEVER goes anywhere alone. She always wanted to see a familiar face in the crowd, so I went with her to her talks—every one of them.

During the next two years, we gave over 300 community education presentations to anyone who would listen. I'd coordinate the times and venues and Dixie would do the talking. Civic groups, church groups, garden clubs, women's groups, chemical plant employees, Rotarians and Rotary Anns, no one was turned down. Most were small groups, twenty or thirty people.

Dixie's name and breast cancer became synonymous throughout the community and women started insisting on having her as their doctor. Going with her to all those talks was a great education for me. She also took me to physician conferences, and I soon learned the jargon and realized that seldom did the doctors agree about the different methods of screening or ways to treat cancer. It was no wonder that women got confused if they heard one thing from one doctor and another thing from the next one.

During all those community talks, the trips we took together, and especially the many Saturdays we spent sunbathing in her pool, Dixie and I became friends and we dreamed of the future.

It was at one of those conferences that we met Rose Kushner. Rose worked for the *Baltimore Sun* and was the first female journalist to cover Vietnam; she stood about five feet tall, was very proud of her Jewish heritage, and had a way of 'telling it like it was,' no matter the consequences. She was my hero.

When Rose found the lump in her breast she went to a surgeon who told her he would do the biopsy, saying, "It is probably nothing. After all, eighty percent of the time these lumps are benign." He told her that when she was on the operating table, if it was cancer, he would just tell Harvey, her husband, and do the mastectomy.

"Why are you telling Harvey?" she demanded, "These are my breasts!"

The doctor argued with her, explaining that there was no need for her to undergo anesthesia twice, once for the biopsy and then a second time for the mastectomy. "Besides," he repeated, "it's probably nothing."

At that time, it was standard procedure to keep a woman under anesthesia, remove the lump, and if it was cancer, remove the entire breast.

Rose was appalled at the idea that a woman could wake up and find her breast gone. She sure wasn't going to have that happen to her! But she had to talk to sixteen surgeons before she found one who would wake her up and let her make the decision. Of course, it turned out to be cancer.

That experience launched her work in breast cancer education. She wrote a book entitled *Why Me? What Every Woman Should Know About Breast Cancer to Save Her Life,* one of the few books written for lay people outlining treatment plans, explaining tests such as ER/PR receptor testing, one test women needed to insist on having. Back then everyone received the same chemotherapy, no matter if it worked or not. When her book was published in 1979, having the word "breast" in the title meant the book was sequestered in the back storage rooms of bookstores and women had to ask for it. Rose was forced to change the title to *Alternatives.*

Reading her book, I understood more than I ever had from listening to the physicians. So imagine how excited I was when I saw her name listed as one of the speakers at the International Breast Cancer Conference that Dixie and I were attending in Miami. I wrote her a letter, applauding her work and asking if she'd meet with us sometime during the conference. I was hoping she'd agree to coffee, but she wrote back saying she had an evening free for dinner and would we join her?

I could barely contain myself on that sparkling March evening in Miami, when Dixie and I sat in a five star restaurant with the famous Rose Kushner and her husband Harvey. The meal was lost to the conversation. I had watched her earlier that day, totally in awe of her knowledge and ability as she debated Dr. Bernie Fisher, one of the leading authorities on breast cancer, about patient rights. At dinner, listening to her talk, it was obvious that she knew every medical whiz in the breast cancer field, as well as every congressman on Capitol Hill. She had strong views on most everything and was more than willing to share them.

At one point during dinner, Dixie was telling her about all the community presentations she had done in the last year, which only solicited a scowl from Rose. She obviously wasn't impressed.

"I used to do that," she said, "and like you, I did it for free. I would go anywhere, anytime, gave hundreds of talks. But I learned very quickly that my time has value and people appreciate you more when you charge something." Then she went on to say, "Besides, all those speeches don't mean squat. A few women hearing about early detection won't make any difference. Until screening mammograms are covered by Medicare, it doesn't matter how much educating you do."

She argued that the only way to make any real change in the world is through the legislative process. Once Medicare covered mammograms, private insurance companies would follow suit. I could sense that Dixie was bristling at Rose's comment "speeches don't mean squat," but she maintained her poise and continued talking about how important it was for women to know about mammography.

Rose leaned forward, "And then what, Dixie? What happens after they hear about it, where do they go to have one?" she challenged.

"That's just it! That's what I'm saying," Dixie exclaimed, "I convinced the administrator to lower the price of mammograms. I got him down to eighty bucks but it's still too much. In Houston mammograms cost $160 to $200. Women can't afford that. So many women are coming to me with late stage cancer. It's awful." Dixie talked about her latest case. I knew she was expecting a tad bit of sympathy and neither of us expected Rose's reply.

Rose leaned even deeper into Dixie's space, and said, "Dixie, quit your pissing and moaning. Why don't you get off your ass and do something about it?"

Dixie sputtered and asked, "Like what?"

"Start your own clinic. Create a non-profit. Find a way to take care of those women." Rose launched into a tirade about what could be done if we had any gumption at all.

Looking back, I have no idea what we expected her to say. Maybe we thought she would pat us on the head and tell us we were doing a great job. We came back to Houston with our tails between our legs, feeling whipped. That's when it started. Every Friday, Rose would call me and ask, "What have you done about starting your non-profit?"

I'd say, "Nothing."

The next week she'd call and ask me if I had contacted my congressman about the Medicare bill.

I'd say, "No." My voice seemed to get smaller each time she called.

Every Friday, the call came. "What have you done?" she asked, and my feeble responses never satisfied her.

What I wanted to say was, "I'm working 55-60 hours a week at my regular hospital job, plus doing everything I can to get this non-profit going. Isn't that enough?"

When we finally did receive our non-profit status, I sent a letter to Rose telling her the good news and that we were naming our organization The Rose as a living tribute to her.

Dixie's married name at that time was Rose, my maiden name was Rose, and we'd met Rose Kushner. What WERE we going to call this place? We sure didn't want it to be the Breast Cancer Institute of Texas! What we did want was a name that was inviting, a name that conveyed it was a place made for women; a name they would come to trust.

When Rose received my letter, naturally, she called me. "What the hell do I need a living tribute for?" she demanded. At the time, I was mortified, but today I have to laugh whenever I think of that. There was just no way I would ever PLEASE that woman!

Back in the conference room, the new employees were also laughing at my story. I opened the black notebook and held up a photograph of Dixie and Rose taken in 1984. "This is Rose, can't you see the feistiness in her?" I put the notebook down, and said, "Unfortunately, Rose never saw either of our centers. She died in 1991 from a reoccurrence. But later Harvey told me that whenever she gave a talk, and she gave a lot of them, she always managed to work in the fact that there was this place in Houston, Texas named after her."

I smiled, looked down at the picture and then back up at the group. "I love telling the story of Rose because we all need to have a Rose in our life, someone who can believe for us what we can't believe for ourselves. Everyone has a dream or has something they feel passionate about. It's the Roses of the world who care enough to push us, who insist we turn our dreams into a reality." I paused, and added, "And if we aren't the ones with the dream, then we need to be a Rose and be the one doing the pushing."

Heads nodded. My time was almost over. I could tell they were getting restless and ready for lunch.

"Before we break for lunch I want to share one more story with you. Part of my job at Bayshore Hospital was also being the medical photographer. I took a lot of pictures in the operating room. The patient was always draped, and many times my only thought was off-setting the bright lights and using the correct f-stop. But when Dixie called asking me to bring my camera to her office, I knew I wasn't going to have to worry about f-stops or lighting.

"I knew from the smell that permeated through the exam room door, I was about to see something no one should ever see or ever have to experience. Even today, nothing ever prepares me for seeing advanced stage breast cancer."

I opened the notebook and held up a picture of a woman's torso, taken from just under her chin to her waist. Everyone in the room gasped. Some turned their faces away or covered their mouths with their hands.

In the picture, one breast was firm and youthful appearing, the other breast looked like something had exploded right out of it. A huge, sickish yellow, cauliflower-looking swelling of flesh and blood formed an open gaping cavern. It was larger than a man's fist and totally encompassed the breast, consuming the space where the nipple had once been. Peering into the cavern of flesh, the muscles covering her ribcage could be seen.

"This woman was Hispanic, a single mother with two kids and no money. She had to keep working for as long as possible. She didn't know there was anywhere to go without insurance, and back then there wasn't. She was dead within two weeks of this picture being taken."

I flipped the notebook over to the next picture.

"This woman was 42 years old and had kept her condition hidden for two years. Her husband had lost his job and insurance. She didn't want it to be a pre-existing condition. At first it was just a small lump, then it grew and finally erupted through the skin. She kept it covered with diapers to absorb the seepage."

In the picture, a big raw hunk of tissue, looking like a couple of pounds of hamburger meat with liquid stuff oozing from it, was sitting on the outside of the woman's breast. A closer look and it was obvious that the 'hunk' was coming from the inside of her body, stretching the skin in a grotesque shape with part of a nipple left clinging to the bloody mixture of flesh.

The group shifted in their seats, one employee had tears running down her face.

"Back then I was so young, so naïve. I couldn't believe she had walked around with this for two years. I asked Dixie, 'How in the world could she have kept this hidden from her husband?'

"Dixie's reply was kind. 'Dorothy,' she said, 'her husband was out of work for a long time, they are going to lose their home. They're broke with three kids to feed. These are hard times. People aren't intimate when things get that bad.'

"Even at this stage, this woman thought she could have surgery and treatment, but the truth was the only thing that could be done was to hold her hand while she died."

Slowly, I looked deep into each person's eyes around the table while asking, "Can you imagine her worry during those two years? Her fear? Being so alone, not being able to tell anyone? I took pictures of thirteen women who looked like this or worse during those first two years."

The room was quiet. I added, "Harris County Hospital still sees a woman like these women every month; here at The Rose, we see one every quarter."

A technologist nodded, she knew what I meant. She'd seen women in the same shape and she knew about the smell of rotting flesh.

I looked around the room at the faces of our new employees, the people who would welcome and help and comfort and guide our patients. And I thought about the conference call with the board that was scheduled after lunch. I couldn't imagine losing The Rose. I couldn't imagine leaving those 33,000 people alone in a system that didn't care for them.

I closed the binder and tapped it with my index finger. "Until we no longer see women like these," I said, "our work isn't done."

Chapter 2
Endowing A Dream

It was ten minutes after seven when Dixie called me on that rainy morning in June, 1986.

"Dorothy, are you watching *The Today Show*?" Her words were quick, she was out of breath, and before I could answer, she went on, "There was a story about a prize, an award, it's called Make Your Dream or something like that. $100,000 goes to the winner. Dorothy, this could be it! Our answer!" There was a pause over the line, then she added with authority, "I have a feeling about this one."

I groaned; another one of those Dixie feelings. But, I reminded myself, *Every once in a while they pan out*. "Slow down, Dixie," I ordered, "an award? What was the name of it again?"

"Something about dreams, and it will go to people who want to do something good but don't have the money to make it happen." She read off the number and I wrote it down.

"I'm late for my rounds," she said, "but call them." The phone clicked off.

The award turned out to be Endow A Dream, sponsored by philanthropist millionaire Clements Stone. Dixie had been right about the amount: $100,000 would allow the winner to fund their dream. I called the organization and they promised to send the application.

Unfortunately, the one critical piece of information that Dixie didn't hear was the requirement that organizations must be a non-profit 501(c)3. Nine months before, in October, 1985, I had filed a DBA (doing business as) for The Rose. I had found people to serve on the governing board and we met irregularly, mainly to talk about the need to receive our non-profit status.

But if we wanted to apply for this award, it was time the talking stopped. The deadline was only thirteen days away.

Somehow, we found a lawyer who was willing to file the paperwork. Michael probably thought we were crazy setting up a non-profit that offered low cost mammograms. He made us explain and re-explain what it was we wanted to do. Although our charity work has always been significant at The Rose, we didn't base our application on providing free services. In fact, from the very beginning we emphasized that those who could afford to pay for services would, allowing us to care for those who could not.

If Michael didn't think the business model was crazy enough, he sure questioned our sanity when we told him we needed it prepared, sent to the Feds (IRS), and approved in less than two weeks. Part of the application process required obtaining a state charter, plus submitting Articles of Incorporation with the state and a complete budget for the next four years.

But he agreed to help. Dixie and I shared the cost of his fee, a whopping $1,300. I put in $400 and she put in the rest. It was a real investment for both of us. Her divorce had strapped her cash flow and my husband was unemployed, that 400 bucks was the last of my personal savings.

The next week was spent rounding up facts and figures, and every evening I worked on writing the narrative and producing a budget. I was also crafting the award application and it had a ton of its own requirements.

When the non-profit application was finished, Michael started hand-carrying it through the filing process. Seven days later, on August 19, 1986, we were notified of the approval of our non-profit status with a back-dating to July 31, 1986. The Rose was finally official! It was Miracle Number One and a portent of events to come.

We didn't win the Endow A Dream award. But we finally had the legal form showing that The Rose was a non-profit. That piece of paper and some big dreams were about all we had, except for some great publicity. I kept churning out news releases, setting up television and radio interviews, and nominating Dixie for awards. One nomination paid off big time. Dixie was selected as one of the top ten Women on the Move, her story and this dream of opening a place called The Rose dominated half a page of the *Houston Post*, in color no less. Back in the mid-'80s that was significant coverage.

Some of the Bayshore doctors grumbled about all the publicity she was receiving—especially the new cardiologist, who couldn't understand how the hospital's breast center and its breast surgeon were getting more attention than his open heart surgery program. "I hold a human heart in my hand, watch it beat, and put it back again," he boasted. "Lopping off breasts can't compare to that."

The radiologists were almost as annoyed and continued to whine about Dixie, a general surgeon, looking at mammograms. Dixie wasn't reading them, but she insisted that her patients bring their studies with them for clinical correlation. She wanted to see on the films what she was feeling with her hand.

When The Rose became a non-profit, the grumbling turned into outright complaints and subtle accusations that anything I was doing to promote Dixie and The Rose was a conflict of interest. Somehow I skirted most of the issues, mainly because the hospital administrator had a lot bigger fish to fry.

But our friend Joyce didn't fare as well. As the director of radiology, she managed the hospital's breast center. She was the person who had stood by Dixie during the equipment debate with the administrator. For her to be involved in starting up this non-profit (perceived by the radiologists as direct competition to the hospital), was professional suicide. Joyce had over 25 years of service and was looking forward to retirement, and none of the grief I got from the medical staff could ever compare to the political tightrope she walked daily.

I always said I had the very best job in the hospital. My work in public relations spanned the gamut from news releases to press conferences, coordinating galas for 500 doctors and their spouses, and managing volunteers. Occasionally, a late night call meant a return trip to the hospital because of an explosion at one of the nearby chemical plants. Those were the sad, intense times, when hysterical families would be lining the halls waiting for word while the media would be in my face with their demands. But those times were rare, and, for the most part, I absolutely loved my job.

There was a lot of good natured teasing among the directors, and we managed to work in times of play, with me orchestrating hundreds of employee events. For Go Texan Days, I wrote and directed a play each year featuring our doctors in a Bayshore version of the television series *Gunsmoke*. The employees went wild seeing their favorite physicians and directors acting out some hokey scene as Marshall Dillon or Black Bart or Miss Kitty, with Baby Face Williams thrown in. Everyone decked out in denim, cowboy boots and hats. The Holidays were the best times, with directors showing up at 5 a.m. to distribute frozen turkeys out of the back of a refrigerated truck to the night shift employees. They all worked throughout the day, griping about frost-bitten fingers and announcing I really 'owed' them this time.

Most of all it was the '80s, a time when folks—especially our Bayshore crew—took off for happy hour at the drop of a hat and weekend Trivial Pursuit games went on until 2 and 3 o'clock in the morning. I had a brand new home in a newly developed subdivision, and our house became the weekend 'go to' place. Its open design spilled out onto the backyard patio and was perfect for parties. Folks would potluck it or we'd grill, my job was being the hostess, hubby's was cooking. During that first year of home ownership, there were only two weekends when we didn't entertain.

But that camaraderie changed almost overnight when managed healthcare reared its ugly head. Suddenly the hospital administrator was gone, along with a few others, and rumors of layoffs ran amuck. By the time The Rose became an official non-profit, the hospital was undergoing a transition to new ownership and the turf wars between Dixie and the radiologists had grown fierce. Employee morale was at an all-time low and the hospital's reputation suffered.

I was working so hard at the hospital and The Rose that I didn't have time to think. I was the lowest paid director at the hospital and I knew I should be worried; my job was on the line as much as Joyce's. Those house payments were high and my husband was out of work again.

But silly me, I continued to dream and plot with Dixie about The Rose and hammered away at my day job. It wasn't until Joyce talked a guy named Ron Smith into donating a machine to us that big things started to happen.

He was the owner of an imaging service, and when he donated a fully dedicated mammography GE imaging system—$160,000 worth of equipment—our dream leapfrogged closer to reality. It was January of 1987, and we finally had a machine. The only problem was that we didn't have a place to put it and we knew we couldn't possibly afford the staff to run it or pay for film or chemical supplies.

Weekends were spent with Dixie and me scouting out possible locations for The Rose. She was like one of those early pioneers walking around with a divining rod looking for water. We would pull up to a shopping center; she'd get out, and walk around, then say, "Nope, not it!" and hop back into the truck. We had lots of options to explore—hundreds of vacant office buildings were another fallout of the bad economy of the '80s.

Finally, we came across South Green Shopping Center, at Fuqua and the Gulf Freeway. We both liked something about that spot, which started looking even better after the leasing agent said we could have a space for free for the first three months and after that he'd charge us $3 for every paying woman we screened. We thought it was a heck of a deal, but then what did we know?

We soon learned that we could be kicked out of the space at the drop of a hat when a real tenant with a signed lease came along. During those first six months, The Rose was moved three times, and each time it meant moving equipment and furniture and reprinting letterhead, expenses we could ill afford. By the time move three was forced upon us, we smartened up and actually signed a three-year lease.

There were a lot of things we didn't know then, especially about radiology. If we hadn't had Joyce involved in those early days, working right beside us, The Rose never would have opened. After she won over Ron and secured the machine, she set up our licenses and ensured our approval from the state. She even recruited Terry, her very best technologist, to come to work for us, and sweet-talked her own family members into volunteering at the center. After a while though, the pressure at the hospital made it clear that she had to make a choice. It was a sad day for me when she resigned and left us on our own.

Dixie knew everything about breast cancer and 'doctoring' and I knew a bunch about 'public relationing,' but we had a whole lot to learn about non-profiting. Neither of us had a clue about the technical side of running an imaging center and fundraising was alien to both of us.

It's difficult to admit that our first fundraiser involved auctioning off men, but it's true. The Bachelor of Distinction event was held at the local Hilton Hotel, and a local group of business women, the Soroptimists, were our volunteers. It was a modest affair, the hotel even allowed us to bring in snacks.

Popular news celebrity, Kathryn Turner, emcee for the night, said she had never seen anyone as frightened as Dixie was with being on stage. Dixie wore a fancy evening dress from Shirley's Bridal Shop and, with Sherry commandeering the event, we crossed into the wild wonderful world of special events. Helping her collect the money, distribute the food, and handle the bar were leading business women from the community: Rosalie, Stella, and Robbie. Those women, along with other Soroptimists, would host annual events for The Rose until 2005.

We auctioned off 'dates' with 29 bachelors: physicians, bankers, lawyers, even a professional wrestler and an ex-husband or two. The women were bidding on a night out with their favorite picks and it was all for a good cause. The top winning bachelor, at $500, was none other than Dr. Alan 'Baby Face' Williams, the area's favorite OB/GYN. Dixie's ex-husband ran a close second.

As bad as it was to be auctioning off men, what I wore that night—a skimpy female Tuxedo outfit with dark silky hose and high heels—was worse. I must have been out of my mind. But we raised $7,000! It was a fortune to us, and the seed money that allowed us to open our first screening center.

Whenever someone tells me their group is too small to make a difference in the world, I tell them the story of the Bachelors Auction and the handful of women who believed in us. They didn't know then that every snack they donated, every hour they spent addressing and mailing invitations, and every decoration they hauled in to transform that huge ballroom into a magical place would mean a chance at life for thousands of women in the future.

Chapter 3
The Early Years
1987-1989

So there we were, with money in hand, an office space rented, and on October 15, 1987, The Rose Mammography Center opened with a waiting list of sixty women. The cost of a mammogram was only $50 and we offered a sponsorship program to high-risk women who couldn't afford to pay. Everything in the center had been donated, from furniture to filing cabinets to the pictures on the walls. Our décor was 'early garage sale,' but the volunteers made it seem homey, the medical care was excellent, and the women felt comfortable.

The entire center only occupied 980 square feet. About a third was devoted to the reception area, a tiny sliver of a room at the very back end of the space created the staff lounge, and the rest housed the mammography equipment. There was a huge round pole that stood smack dab in the middle of the reception area. We tried to camouflage it with plants and coat trees but it never cooperated. It was still a big fat ugly pole that got in the way. When guest speakers came to talk to our newly organized breast cancer support group, they had to weave around that pole while doing presentations. The crowd of survivors and family members would sway from one side to the other, trying to see either the slides or the speaker. Watching people squirm, first raising up, then crouching down, and finally moving back and forth was like being in a funhouse with those mirrors.

But the speakers came anyway, especially Dr. Haq, an oncologist who once apologetically described chemotherapy as using an "atomic bomb" to get rid of a wart. The type of chemotherapy treatment used in the mid-'80s was just short of being lethal; personalized medicine was still decades away. The saying "if the cancer doesn't kill you, the treatment probably will" was a common one. But Dr. Haq did what he had to do to help women stay alive, and he made the last day of a woman's chemotherapy treatment a celebration, presenting his patients with red roses and hugs. He was one of our heroes.

We were pretty proud of our center, especially the two donated bookcases that had once been built for a lawyer's office. They were huge, over eight feet tall, and when pushed together made a temporary wall and created a visual divide for the high ceilings and long narrow space. They were so heavy that it took five guys to move them into place. We positioned them four feet away from the lone real wall that separated the reception area from the imaging area. The arrangement created a tiny alcove wide enough to fit in a desk.

Those bookshelves and everything else in the center were soon covered with a layer of light blue dust from the Xerox film. It was part of the mammography processing system, any center that did mammograms fought it, but for us getting rid of the blue became a personal daily battle.

But in spite of it all, patients came and we were open for business. It would be another two years before that five by eight foot alcove nestled behind those bookshelves would become my office, but in the meantime I did what I had to as The Rose's executive director.

Remembering the people who took those first steps with us still makes me smile. From the beginning, volunteers were the heart of The Rose, and Anna Belle was one of those people.

She, like almost all of the employees during that first five years, started as a volunteer. She was a patient of Dixie's, having gone through her own bout with breast cancer a few years earlier. Breast cancer was the nemesis of her family, her paternal aunt and two of her sisters had died from it, another sister was currently fighting it. Dixie had never seen breast cancer coming down the father's side with such a vengeance.

Meeting Anna Belle meant coming face to face with the human side of this insidious disease. Breast cancer was no longer a clinical diagnosis confined to a few women who briefly crossed my path; it became fully exposed, unfathomable in its callousness. Its true destructive force, its very existence, mocked a woman's life and her body. The threat of reoccurrence was palpable and became a silent and invisible intruder bordering every conversation, every success, every passage of normal living.

Anna Belle would have violently objected to that description. She'd insist that breast cancer was just one of those things that happen in a person's life. "Everyone goes through something," she'd say. But I watched too many times as breast cancer chopped away at all the corners of her being and I knew the impact it had on her family.

It is difficult to describe Anna Belle. Take everything good and mix it with a lot of country, top it with genuine hospitality, weave in some of the most outrageous off-colored humor you'd ever expect to find in a woman, and you'd have a glimpse of her. A real natural beauty, she had a certain elegant presence about her that was accented by many layers of denim. Anna Belle told it as it was, and sometimes the telling wasn't easy to hear.

You'd think someone who had such an intimate history with breast cancer would be incredibly sympathetic to the plight of others, but she wasn't. She never had any truck with whiners. Her approach was "You do what you have to do, pay attention, and don't believe everything the doctors tell you!" She insisted that she was the only one in her life who got to decide how long she was going to live.

She always had a new joke to share. Invariably it bordered on the risqué or bawdy but would be just clean enough to squeak by. She'd fall into hysterical laughter when she delivered the punch line and I couldn't help but join in, her humor was infectious.

It was Anna Belle's spunk that greeted our first patients. She'd make an appointment over the phone with a new patient, and then hang up saying, "That one will never find us."

She maintained a theory that half of our patients were geographically challenged, she never said which half, and the only way to get them through the doors was to give them a food landmark. "We're in the strip center across from Chili's," she'd tell them, or "We're just down from TGI Friday's." She reasoned that everyone should know the location of these two monuments to culinary excellence and providing patients with the names of cross streets or our actual address was just a waste of time.

I was still working at Bayshore and spending weekends and weeknights managing payroll, paying bills, grant writing, and sending news releases out for The Rose, but I met with Anna Belle once a week for lunch. She probably worked more hours than anyone, and always without complaint. Work back then was dusting those blue-covered shelves, vacuuming floors, washing and drying the patient cover-ups, as well as answering phones, making appointments, being the receptionist, money handler, and intake person. In that role, she had no patience with any woman who failed to complete her profile properly.

"Can you believe this?" she snapped, pushing the clipboard at me and pointing to the paperwork on it. "This woman said she had never had breast surgery, but then she says right underneath it that she has implants! How the heck does she think they got there?" She would wave toward a pile of patient forms on her desk, "Tell me, how is it that nobody knows when they last saw their doctor or had their periods? Don't these people have calendars?" The ultimate outrage for her was women who lied about their age on the patient information sheets, "That lady hasn't seen fifty in years. Who does she think she's kidding?"

But she was never more vocal than when she thought someone was trying to take advantage of our sponsorship program—the tiny fund we had managed to raise that covered the cost of a woman who didn't have the $50 to pay for her mammogram. I don't think any non-deserving person managed to get by her. She'd look the patient right in the eyes and make a comment about what a nice suit or ring she had on (or fine automobile she was driving), and then immediately ask how much she thought she could pay towards this mammogram.

I worried about her questioning the patients too much and wrestled with the thought that we might actually turn away someone who really needed our help. As it turned out, my worries were unfounded. When someone was really down on her luck, Anna Belle would be the first in line to help. She truly had a heart of gold, and that was never more obvious than during the support groups.

In 1989, the jury was still out concerning the clinical and/or psychological value of support groups. Survivors often thought, *I have my family or friends to lean on, I don't need a support group*, and, of course, most of the physicians thought it was the shy side of voodoo.

But Dixie was convinced that nothing was more important than The Rose offering a support group to breast cancer survivors. And her ideas were vindicated when Dr. David Spiegel's original report on the "Effect of psychosocial treatment on survival of patients with metastatic breast cancer" was published in *Lancet* in October of 1989. In essence, it reported that women who participated in support groups experienced twice the survival rate as those who didn't.

During those first few months, the only women who attended the group were Dixie's patients, but before long, physicians from all over the community were recommending our support group to their patients.

Dixie's patients definitely had the advantage. She always suggested her newly diagnosed women attend a support group meeting prior to their surgery. She didn't make it a requirement, she simply convinced them that they could learn what to expect from other women who'd had a mastectomy or lumpectomy.

Most women struggling with receiving a life and death sentence had enough to sort through and they sure didn't expect what they found at our support group. It had been christened The Rose Garden and met every second and fourth Tuesday at the center. We would push the two particle board desks against the wall and move the mismatched orange and green chairs next to the overstuffed brilliant blue couch to create a makeshift semicircle.

First-timers entered a room packed with women who were

obviously at different stages of treatment, some were bald, some were not, some were old, some were young, a few had family members with them. The first impression of The Rose Garden was the sound of laughter floating over the din of talking, punctuated by the smells of fresh coffee and sweet food.

The socializing didn't let up until Dixie arrived. She usually ran late, but no one cared. Then, as now, Dixie brought hope into the room.

The meeting would unofficially begin with Anna Belle distributing copies of breast cancer related articles and talking about what new books were available from our lending library. The prized document for every first-timer was Dr. Dixie Melillo's Official Vitamin List. You can't imagine the criticism Dixie received from colleagues because she recommended vitamins. She always countered with "What could it hurt?" A few years later every vitamin that appeared on her list was being recommended by the leading cancer institutions. She also questioned the dangers of hormone replacement therapy and, sure enough, about ten years later, all her concerns and more were validated.

Once the meeting began, we'd go around the room, with each woman introducing herself and sharing a little information about her journey.

Teresa wore a long red wig that looked like it was way too much hair for her body, a body that seemed to get tinier at each meeting. "I'm Teresa, and one week after I turned 32 years old, I was diagnosed. That was thirteen months ago." Her skin was pale and her freckled face looked sad. I tried to imagine her smiling, something I hadn't seen her do since she started attending the group. "I'm taking my last chemotherapy this week. I have a nine-year-old who ignores everything and a three-year-old who wants to know where Mommy's hair went."

Nancy was next; her dark hair was cropped close to her head, her body swollen. Her short stature emphasized the extra weight. "I'm Nancy, and I was diagnosed two years ago but had a reoccurrence. I've got mets to the liver and I've done the rounds of chemo, so the next step is having a bone marrow transplant. It all depends on if everything works out, the insurance approves it, and if my blood count comes back okay." Her movements were deliberate and there was a cautious sense about her, as if she didn't want to touch anything or anyone. There was sharpness to her eyes and in her speech. The group understood that the cancer had spread to her liver and her immune system was compromised, a common cold could easily escalate, the mildest infection could turn into certain death.

Charlie was in her mid-fifties. She had an easy smile, her round face and manner reminded me of everyone's grandmother. "I'm Charlie, and this is my second round with it also. Chemotherapy just isn't working. I had a double mastectomy." Charlie's daughters always came with her; they were in their late twenties. They sat on either side of her and, straight-faced, would tell the group that their mother was really being terribly grumpy lately and they had to ignore her. The new folks in the group would gasp or look shocked. They would continue with "After all, she does have the big C." It didn't take long before we all realized their talk was part of a gentle teasing between the three women. Maybe it was the way the young women looked at their mom, or the way they held her hand, there was a magic between them and their love was palpable.

"I'm Karen, and like Teresa, I was 32 when I had my mastectomy on the right side. A year after my diagnosis, I had to have a mammogram on the other side, this was before The Rose opened, so I went somewhere else to have it." She nodded at me knowingly. I smiled back. Karen was one tough cookie. Her attire was simple, jeans and a plaid shirt, no nonsense. Her square shoulders begged for someone to knock the chip off and her in-your-face way of talking actually baited folks. It was no secret that she held most of the medical establishment in disdain. "Well, when I got there I found out that the lady at the desk had cancelled my appointment. I was livid! She said, 'You're too young to have a mammogram.' I just looked at her and fired back, "Well, Lady, I'm not too young to have breast cancer!'" We all shook our heads.

"I'm Mary, and I haven't had my surgery yet," said the next woman, and the room became quiet. "I just learned about my diagnosis yesterday." Mary was in her forties, her teased brown hair formed a perfect helmet around her face, her eyes were bright with fear, yet her words were measured and soft. It was clear she was finding this discussion a bit too public.

Someone began asking the standard questions to get her talking. Was Dixie her doctor? A nod, and the stories started tumbling out about what it was like to be a patient of Dixie's. They'd tell her she was now part of a community that no one would volunteer to be in, but at least with Dixie as the doctor, it was tolerable. They talked and assured her and each other that they'd make their thirtieth reunion.

Someone else shared her own surgery experience, explaining that she had stopped being afraid the moment she was taken down to the operating suite and saw Dixie waiting on her. "Dixie walked alongside me while they wheeled me through those big double doors. She held my hand all the way into the operating room. She's the last face you see when you go to sleep and the first one you see when you wake up.

She'll get you through this."

Everyone always clapped when the gorgeous, well-coifed woman wearing the prettiest clothes in the world announced, "I'm Ola Mae, and I'm a thirteen-year survivor." For the newbies, meeting someone who had managed to outrun the enemy was the highlight of the evening. But most of us were more interested in hearing about Ola Mae's new boyfriend or her latest travel adventure than her triumph over cancer. Her shiny silver locks confirmed she was pushing sixty but her spirit and energy rivaled any twenty-year-old, so did her figure. She was petite and incredibly shapely. She never went anywhere without her makeup, her full lips were bright red, her skin creamy smooth, and her bejeweled glasses made her eyes even bigger. She was the ultimate volunteer, busy with a dozen organizations from Eastern Star to MD Anderson and The Rose. Her only problem was not having enough hours in the day to do all she was scheduled to do.

By this time Anna Belle was clearing her third cancer-free year. She had undergone a double lumpectomy; the second one was done about five months after her first surgery. She was one of the rare women who didn't lose her hair during chemotherapy, something she usually didn't share with the group. She had lots of other stories to share.

It was fascinating the way the focus of the group's conversation usually moved away from diagnosis or ideas to make treatment more bearable (always wear a cotton shirt during radiation or use this medicine when the sores break out in the mouth) to more personal issues. Somehow the group always got around to talking about what they had learned and how they were establishing new priorities, sometimes on a daily basis.

One woman shared how guilty she felt because she didn't babysit the grandchildren anymore. She was too tired from the chemotherapy. "Good!" pronounced Dixie, "Tell your kids they can find another babysitter. They may even have to pay for it, but they'll find one, I guarantee you. But also tell them they won't be able to find another grandmother!"

Another woman said she wasn't being a good wife since she couldn't keep up with all the household chores. The others dove in on that one. "Let it pile up!" they said, "Get that good-for-nothing husband of yours to help!"

There would be the occasional skittish talk of what else a "good wife" didn't feel like doing or how unattractive they felt at times, but usually those stories got a little too uncomfortable and just hung in the air, seldom resolved.

A very few dared to talk of their bitterness. There was never any judgment from those listening. Those who were brave enough to share their own regrets encouraged the others to talk out their feelings. It was okay to be mad or sad or depressed, but the group had a way of not letting anyone dwell in the mire of despair for too long.

I realize now what kind of emotional courage it really took for those women sitting around in those mismatched chairs to approach death while still so alive. So many in our group were dealing with a reoccurrence or with cancer at a stage well beyond the help of conventional medicine. The unspoken undertow that kept the group going forward was the collective severity of the illness.

A few would share how they were learning to put their needs first and were taking better care of themselves. Some would tell of a friend's kindness, a meal cooked, a relative who came and collected the kids and took them away for a weekend.

Two of the women with metastatic cancer talked of their progress in creating their personal home movies for the future. They'd describe writing their scripts and talking into the camera, telling their children or grandchildren what they might not be around to say at their high school graduation or on their wedding day.

Dixie told everyone that those of us who didn't have breast cancer should have to pay "good money" to attend support group meetings. She would end the meetings saying, "None of us knows how long we have on this earth. This group has taught me that I need to appreciate every sunrise and every sunset. And I've also learned the importance of hugs."

She'd smile and remind everyone, "Hugs are good for the immune system. It's true! There is clinical proof that touching is healing." (She was right again, during the next few years there would be a ton of research proving that human touch stimulates the t-cells and reduces stress levels.) "Besides," she'd continue, "it feels good. You can never get enough hugs."

Dixie would start the rounds, wrapping her arms around the woman nearest to her and moving from one to the other until everyone had been soundly hugged. Reluctantly, the talk and laughter would ebb and a few would linger behind to help clean up. Some nights we got out early. Any time before 10 p.m. was early.

I attended more funerals during those early years than my priest officiated over. It was a tough couple of years.

I was ecstatic that The Rose was finally open, but I could no longer manage those long hours working full time at the hospital and spending every evening and weekend working for The Rose. We couldn't afford a salary for a 'real director' and we sorely needed someone full-time at the helm. It took months of submitting grants before I finally found one to cover a modest salary for six months. I said goodbye to Bayshore and walked away from seventeen years of my life, leaving behind friends, big company benefits, and professional advantages.

But I was happy. My husband was working, I had a beautiful home that I loved, and I was crazy about the possibilities for this place called The Rose.

Little did I know that within the next six months it would all go to hell.

Chapter 4
Toxic

The first time I saw Saucy her nose was pressed against the wire walls of a big cage at a local animal shelter. No matter how much I tried to ignore her, that little dog was determined to get my attention. She climbed over seven or eight other puppies, all intent on bowls of food, to lock her huge front paws into the wire of the cage. The floor of fur moved beneath her and threatened to bounce her off. Her tail thumped against the others and her eyes, black with a hint of blue surrounding the iris, stared at me.

"I didn't want a black dog," I murmured, looking away and into the other cages, "but then this wasn't supposed to be my dog anyway." I don't know where I got the idea that I needed to find a dog for my husband, but it soon became an obsession.

The last eight years of marriage had been bumpy. Alan had trouble keeping a job; things just didn't work for him, physically or mentally. I hadn't known him when the accident happened; he was twenty-nine, on the golf course, and somehow survived being hit by lightning. His family told me about the month he spent in a coma and the year it took him to learn to walk again. They didn't say much else about the accident or what led to his divorce after it, and neither did he.

When I got the dog idea, Alan was in Saudi Arabia on a real long-shot of a business deal. He had been gone for a month. Maybe it was the time alone, maybe it was the growing uneasiness in my soul when I measured the distance between us even when we were in the same room, but whatever it was, I yearned for something else, something alive in my life.

Dixie convinced me that a pet from Special Pals made sense. With a husband whose commission was always iffy and my salary at Bayshore, I sure wouldn't be shelling out three or four hundred dollars for a pure breed dog like she owned—the $35 adoption fee was perfect.

It didn't take long for me to fall in love with that ball of fur after we went to the 'meet and greet' area. It was a small enclosed courtyard surrounding a well-trodden area of dirt and worn down grass. The Special Pals worker explained that the puppy was six weeks old, a female, and the last one of a litter of an "unfortunate" coupling of a full breed Chow and Lab.

The worker gently slid the puppy onto the earth and the moment its paws hit the ground, I froze, certain it was going to run over to me and jump in my lap. Instead, she walked around in a circle, with an almost nonchalant attitude. The sun's bright rays showered her, making her deep, dark black fur gleam with red highlights. The Chow part of her was obvious in her rich, thick and shiny fur, the Lab in her oversized ears that flopped back and forth as she strutted. I watched, intrigued by her independence.

Why, she struts around just like a show dog, I thought. *She has to know she's being watched. She's so sure of herself, she is so…*" I struggled for the right word and she stopped, looking right at me, tail wagging, and I would swear later that a smile crossed her sweet little face. "She's so SAUCY!" I said out loud.

Within a week, I was totally enchanted with her, so I was pretty crushed when Alan returned, took one look at Saucy, and said, "It's just a mutt." It had never occurred to me that he would reject her because she wasn't a pure breed.

After six weeks, Saucy became lethargic. I knew something was wrong, deadly wrong. A rushed trip to the vet confirmed that she was close to dying, so totally dehydrated that she needed to stay overnight for intravenous fluids.

"Was it my fault?" I asked. I feared all the flea baths I had given her were the culprit. "Did they made her ill?" I asked, when I picked her up.

The vet said maybe but probably not. "Sometimes puppies just get sick," he reassured me. It would be two years before we found out the real reason for Saucy's first illness and all the illnesses after that. The years ahead would be filled with steroid shots to alleviate the constant itching and scratching, monthly visits to the vet, and watching her suffer.

After a while Alan warmed up to Saucy, but my in-laws didn't and they made no bones about it during their annual Thanksgiving visit. Saucy was only six months old but already topping out at sixty pounds. She quickly picked up that she wasn't adored by these folks and gave them a wide berth as she moved around the house.

On the Saturday after Thanksgiving, my mother-in-law Mary

Louise and I spent the entire day shopping for her Mother of the Bride dress. That and finishing knitting her new son-in-law's Christmas stocking were the last things she had to do before her youngest daughter's upcoming wedding. We never found her dress that day, but after dinner she spent the evening hard at work on the stocking. Around 9 p.m., with a sigh, she exclaimed, "There! It's done!" She held it up for us to admire.

Saucy lay on the floor a few feet away from her, her head balanced on her front paws, she was unusually sedate as she watched Mary Louise. She had been in that spot all evening; her eyes glued on Mary Louise.

Later we would remark that somehow Saucy knew.

At two o'clock in the morning, a voice called out and I sat straight up in bed. A large body stood at our bedroom door. Silhouetted by the light from the hallway, I could make out his tee-shirt and boxer shorts. "Something is wrong with Mary Louise," Alan's father mumbled, "Your mother is making a strange noise. I can't wake her up."

I had the presence of mind to tell Alan to put Saucy out in the backyard as I yelled out other orders. "Call 911! Unlock the front door!"

I jumped on the bed, crawled over to her jerking body, and realized she wasn't breathing. "Help me get her to the floor," I yelled at his dad, who stood motionless, unable to comprehend anything I was saying. I pulled her arms but I couldn't budge her. Almost as soon as I straddled her and started to push on her chest, I heard the siren. Moments later, medics were bursting through the front door and barreling down the hall.

No son should see what Alan did that night. The EMTs quickly moved her to the dining room, pushing furniture out of the way, and laid her on the floor. They stripped her gown from her chest and started CPR. Her skin was so pale, emphasizing the starkness of her nakedness. She looked fragile, almost breakable, as they pushed again and again at her chest. Her breasts were tiny under the huge hands of the man desperately trying to save her life. When an EMT started an IV in her arm, blood gushed out on the carpet. Another tilted her head back off her chest. A stretcher appeared from nowhere.

We watched, silent, as they lifted her limp body and rolled it onto the hard metal carrier and moved quickly out the front door. Alan and his dad followed.

Three very long hours passed before father and son agreed to take her off life support; she had essentially died at the house. I had already called Alan's four sisters, telling them their mother was in trouble. For the next two hours, I made more calls with this impossibly sad news.

We learned later that the majority of women, nearly 70%, die from their first "apparent" heart attack.

That Holiday seemed to mark the beginning of sad times for our household. As it turned out, our brand new house, the first new home I had ever owned, had been built on a toxic waste dump, contaminated for over thirty years by Monsanto.

The oil waste, full of PBCs, ethyl benzene, vinyl chloride, and other cancer causing agents, had been dumped into huge pits dug out in the ground then covered over with dirt. After a while, the toxic waste migrated through the underground water and into the surrounding 58-acre area. By the time that area was finally declared a Superfund site in 1992, thousands of people had relocated, the elementary school had closed, and all 670 brand new homes in the South Bend subdivision were demolished.

Saucy's plight was mild compared to the families who had children born with defects, missing reproductive organs, and terminally ill, or the women who were diagnosed with thyroid and breast cancer. Three of those women attended our support group.

The Brio Superfund site, as it was called, wasn't the first time Monsanto was sued for damaging the health of residents near its Superfund sites through pollution and poisoning, nor would it be the last. By 2012, it would be associated with eleven active cases and twenty archived sites.

The months ahead were filled with such heartache, but talks of lawsuits and toxic wastes and abandoning the house were beyond my comprehension. I kept resisting until there was no other choice. We finally became a part of the second of three class action suits brought against Monsanto for the Brio site. In the end, our lawyers did the most to prove deliberate negligence by the oil company, but the plaintiffs in our suit received the most modest settlement.

Our legal eagles had advised us to stop paying our mortgage and leave the house. Two-thirds of the subdivision had already moved out. We lived in a ghost town, with yards overgrown and homes boarded up. Children no longer played in the streets and the occasional car usually belonged to some investigator.

Silly as it sounds, especially when there was no way we could have managed two house notes, I really struggled over walking the loan and having a foreclosure against our credit. That stigma eliminated buying another house, so the only option was finding a rental. That task turned out to be a lot harder than I ever imagined. After being in my own home for five years, living in a rental house wasn't appealing. Besides, there weren't many around and virtually no one wanted to rent to someone with a dog, especially not a big dog that was used to being inside.

"But she's so well trained," I tried to explain, exasperated after the ninth denial. "She has been a house dog all her life and I assure you..." The phone clicked, signaling that the landlord had hung up. Tears welled up in my eyes and spilled out over my cheeks.

It isn't fair! I seethed. First, trying to juggle the fact that our health was in danger after years of living on top of a toxic dump, then losing the house, and now having would-be landlords treat us like lowlifes. It was bad enough going through the trial, where we were questioned like criminals by the defendants' lawyers: "Have you ever smoked?" "Lived near chemical plants?" "Taken any drugs?" Innuendos attempted to discredit our testimony and shake us up. We stumbled over the most basic questions. It would be sixteen long months before our credit was restored and we could start to think about living a normal life.

But for now, I had to find a new place to live. With only one week left before my 'home' would be padlocked, I found a place in an older neighborhood located in the shadow of the airport. It was far from perfect, but at least the owner didn't care about renting to folks who had a big dog.

Losing that house marked the beginning of a roller coaster ride of years filled with highs and lows. I will never forget the last day I walked through the empty rooms. I said goodbye to all that I had handpicked and loved—every tile, the totally impractical light blue carpet, and the now towering trees that I had planted in the backyard. All the memories of the past five years flooded over me, the weekends of working in the yard, the parties, the people, the day I brought Saucy home.

It was February, 1989, and the timing of losing our home and becoming an official employee of The Rose collided. I worked at a desk in the little alcove behind the bookcases. Gone were the days of filling out a purchase order for supplies or having telephones that worked or a good computer. It would be years before we even had a computer.

I wrote my grants on an old IBM Selectric typewriter and we kept a log of the patients by hand in one of those black-lined steno notebooks. Anna Belle would carefully label each page with the date and day of week and start numbering the lines. Each patient's name and the amount they paid (or didn't pay) was meticulously recorded. We never destroyed those appointment books.

On a good day we had eight to ten women. On a better day we actually had the schedule booked for a full week.

My justification for finally leaving Bayshore came when The Rose's radiologist convinced me to take over the management of her mobile mammography services. If I didn't know anything about running an imaging center, I sure didn't know anything about mobile units.

It had a good mammography machine on it, but that converted RV was in the shop more than it was out. Its generators never could hold up to a full day of screening. If it wasn't the generators conking out, it was the motor itself. One time I had to have it towed to a site! I didn't dare cancel on that customer again.

Then there was the problem of finding a driver for it. Our part-time technologist refused to drive it. My solution was to convince my cousin Helen to give it a try. Helen was already a volunteer, but this was one time I figured I needed to actually pay her for her time. My plan was simple: she could drive it to and from the sites two days a week, be the intake person, and help the tech out on screening days. After all, she had once driven a school bus, so an RV couldn't be all that different…could it? Boy, was that a mistake.

Helen was in her mid-fifties and still trying to figure out what she wanted to be when she grew up. She had a decade of success in the real estate business but the economic bust of the '80s had pretty much wiped that out. A recent divorce meant she was on her own and every dollar counted. On that fateful day of her employment at The Rose, she was holding down four other jobs—all part time.

Another volunteer, Shelly, had offered to go with Helen. Their plan was to find an open space so Helen could practice driving and parking the RV. I stood at the doorway of the center and watched that old oversized van lumber off, sort of wobbling from one side to the other. Shelly was driving.

Maybe if we hadn't been surprised with an unannounced inspection by the state, the day would not have been so disastrous. The inspector showed up about 10 a.m., smack dab in the middle of one of the busiest days we'd ever had. Patients waiting to be screened filled up the room, volunteers filled up the tiny workspace behind the reception desk, and the inspector filled up my cubby hole of an office with her no-nonsense presence and a long list of questions.

For some reason, the inspector was curious about the child who was helping the volunteers stuff envelopes. That child was Helen's grandchild, Crystal, and she always came to help during spring break. My mind raced ahead, was I violating some state law about using children in the work place? Heck, I was already flustered enough and had spent the past hour producing documents, proving to her that our forms and licenses were up to date and our procedures were in place. Finally satisfied with the paperwork, she started on the list of questions. In the middle of her interrogation, the call came.

Shelly's voice was high and frantic. "The ambulance is on its way," she announced.

"What ambulance?" I asked, imagining a five-car pile-up, with that monster van somehow the cause of it.

"The one coming for Helen. She fell out of the van."

"Fell out of the van? What? How? Is she hurt?"

"I think her back is broken," Shelly said flatly.

"BROKEN?" I responded.

"Look, I have to go. I had to leave her on the ground. I found a pay phone at this Seven Eleven here on Crenshaw and Burke. I called the ambulance, then you, but I need to get back to her…"

"Call me back as soon as you can."

I hung up, only to be greeted with the biggest tear-filled eyes any child could ever have. Little Crystal had appeared at my side, she sort of clutched at me with both hands.

"Is Gram hurt?" she cried. "I want to be with Gram." Tears were now gushing down her face.

Other eyes were glaring at me, the inspector wasn't happy with the interruption and she let me know it.

Between apologizing to the inspector and assuring Crystal that Gram would be all right, I motioned for Anna Belle to take Crystal to the back. I continued to answer the inspector's endless questions, but all the while I was silently praying, *Please God, let Helen be all right. I glanced at the clock. Would this woman ever leave?*

By the time the inspector did leave, cautioning me that we had better keep our records squeaky clean and advising me it would be three weeks before her report was filed, Helen was at the hospital getting a CAT scan of her back.

Later, Shelly told me the full story. They had stopped for gasoline at the Seven Eleven and were going to switch places so Helen could drive. Helen had climbed up into the van, had settled in, adjusted her seat, and was reaching for the door handle to close the door.

That's when she fell.

She didn't realize that the van didn't have running boards. When she reached out to close the door, she automatically stretched out with her left foot, trying to feel for the non-existent running board while her hand kept moving toward the door; naturally, her body followed. She tumbled out of the cab, smack flat on her back. She started to get up, but Shelly, who was in her second year of nurse's training, insisted that Helen shouldn't move. She screamed at Helen, "Your back could be broken!" "You could have a head trauma!" "Who knows what could be messed up!"

"Don't move!" she ordered as they waited for the ambulance.

When she heard Helen moaning, she asked, "Are you in pain?"

Helen, trying hard to accommodate 'Nurse' Shelly's instructions, snorted back at her, "No! But I wish you'd get these damn ants off me."

Thank goodness Helen's back wasn't broken, the overnight hospitalization confirmed that she didn't have a concussion, and besides receiving topical ointment for the hundreds of tiny any bites, she was okay and released.

So ended Helen's first paying job with us. That day also signaled the quickly approaching demise of the mobile unit. A month later the roof sprung a leak and it turned out that the metal frame had become twisted, causing the seams to pop. There was no fixing it. I was happy returning those keys to the radiologist. I promised myself I would find another way to bring in revenue.

As it turned out, the inspector found nothing to report, we'd passed on every level. We learned later that someone from the hospital had filed a complaint. Maybe it was the radiologists or the new administration.

At that point, who called the state didn't matter, I was just thankful we had passed. There were way too many other issues to handle. Funding topped the list. The grant that was supposed to cover my six months of salary was being quickly consumed by other needs. I had to find more funding and fast or The Rose's short life would be over.

There was no respite at the place I now called home. The rental house was dreary and dirty. Why I tried to clean it I'll never know, but I did, hours and hours of scrubbing counters, sinks, bathtubs, floors. I posted signs throughout the house that shouted out in big bold letters: This is TEMPORARY.

Alan's dad came to visit at Christmas, the year after Mary Louise had died. He tried, we tried, but the strain and lingering memories were just too much.

I missed my best friend Hazel, who had met the love of her life and moved off to Australia the year before. This would be the second Holiday without her since 1981. My favorite season of the year was filled with sadness. The new year started with Alan being fired and now we were without medical insurance coverage.

It wasn't the first time I knew what it felt like to not have health insurance or fight off that insidious worry that daily stalked around the edges of one's mind. I was counting on us staying well and accident free. It would be six months before The Rose had enough employees to be eligible to apply for group insurance and another year before we could afford to offer it.

But nothing mattered as much as the work at The Rose. It had become my safe haven, a place I could pretend that I had a little bit of control and could still dream about a future. Even with all the other insane, sad happenings of that year, I'll always remember 1989 for a crazy event that would become a tradition and a lifeline for The Rose for the next three decades.

Chapter 5
The Great Shrimp Boil

The day was more than hot, it was sweltering. Houston in July is always hot and humid, but this was one of those days when stepping outside felt like walking straight into an oven.

I was traveling north on I-45 in my old Plymouth with the AC cranked up to maximum. My clothes were sticking to me and little rivulets of sweat ran down my spine and between my legs. I pushed the hair out of my eyes and patted down the frizzy ends sticking out atop my head. I was a mess and getting more aggravated as I tried to keep up with the caravan of pickup trucks ahead of me. Each truck carried precious cargo—fresh shrimp. As I watched the oversized coolers bounce around in the back of the truck ahead of me, I was sure we had lost our minds.

Every charity relies on fundraising events, most have the usual types—simple barbecues or elegant galas or nice luncheons—something sane, but not The Rose.

Our annual fundraiser meant rounding up five or six people who owned pickup trucks to travel thirty miles south to Kemah and load up on fresh shrimp. We needed a lot of coolers and lots of ice, because it was a whole lot of shrimp. It always took more than one stop to get our total supply; nobody carried or sold all the pounds we needed at one place. I didn't do much lifting or hauling of those ice chests, I went along to sign the checks and, of course, for moral support.

Finally loaded up, water streaming out of those chests as the ice was melting way too fast, we all bounced back into town. Then we sat on the tailgates of those same trucks and started de-heading the little suckers, all 600 pounds of them. If the humidity hadn't already managed to steal our breath away, the smell of that fresh shrimp definitely did.

Out of our minds? Yes. But the fun had just begun. De-heading shrimp was step one.

Next we'd round up another group of volunteers and haul garbage bags and boxes full of more food stuff inside the SPJST Lodge. It was the only place in town big enough to accommodate 1,000 people, and the folks who ran the Lodge agreed to let us use it, but only on a Sunday and only if they ran the bar and took its proceeds and only if we left the place spanking clean.

The Slovanska Podporujici Jednota Statu of Texas Lodge was a massive place, easily covering a city block. It offered a huge dance floor, a commercial kitchen area with oversized stoves, stainless steel counters, and plenty of parking. Best of all, it had a gigantic back hall that opened up to the outside, which was a perfect work space for shucking 500 stalks of fresh corn, cleaning 400 pounds of potatoes, and making up 2,000 little containers of cocktail sauce. That preparation took the entire day.

We would have probably had a barbecue or something equally sane if my husband hadn't won a bass boat. He'd aced a hole in one at the Mickey Gilley Charity Golf Tournament for PADAP, a drug rehab organization. His prize was a brand new micro fifteen-foot bass boat, compliments of Gilley's brother, who owned a marine business. It was a really big deal, his photo accepting the boat from Mickey made all the local papers and even captured a spot on the evening news.

As usual, I was oblivious to his latest golfing excursion, so I was pretty surprised when he came home all excited about winning the boat and how it would be a great fundraiser for The Rose. Actually, I didn't follow his logic, it made more sense to me to just sell it and donate the money. But he kept outlining elaborate schemes for a fabulous fundraiser. He talked about involving local celebrities, getting lots of publicity, hosting a dinner or a gala, his ideas were endless.

I had my hands full trying to run the business, write the grants, and manage the mobile unit program that was going downhill fast. I lay awake many nights praying that pile of junk wouldn't break down the next day. It would be another four months before we abandoned that program. But at the time Alan won the boat I was buried in the middle of all of that day-to-day chaos, and pulling together a fundraising event wasn't high on my list.

About a month passed and I still didn't have a clue what to do with that boat. Alan was getting more and more huffy over my apparent lack of interest. That was when I had this dream. It had been one of those fitful nights spent staring at the ceiling worrying over the unit, hoping we'd make payroll and wondering how to find funding. Finally sleep came and with it a magical dream.

I was in a house of ill repute or some sort of similar activity, standing on the mezzanine level, looking down over a room filled with women in waiting. A man entered. Obviously he was a fisherman; he was a big attractive man with a white beard that covered his face. He went up to one of the women and started talking. She was the prettiest woman there and wore the sexiest clothes, tight pants with a sheer top. Her laughter floated up as they started up the stairs.

I woke up knowing that somehow everything would be all right.

That evening, one of the newer couples came to the support group meeting. They'd attended one or two times before but I didn't know them well. During the announcements, I explained that Alan had donated this boat to The Rose but I couldn't figure out how to use it to raise money.

Jim jumped in and said, "What you need is a shrimp boil to go along with the boat theme. I know some folks who could do the cooking!"

His wife Marsha caught his excitement and exclaimed, "Raffle that boat off, sell tickets for $5 each!"

Five dollars? A piece? That amount caused a big debate within the group.

The pros and cons went back and forth until Marsha stopped all the chatter by saying, "We won't have a bit of trouble selling tickets at that price, just give them to Jim and me."

I remember staring at her and thinking how sexy she looked. She was so attractive, a big busted woman with long dark hair, and her oversized blouse hit just the right spot at the top of her leggings. Her treatment had just started.

She and Jim exchanged glances. They loved to party and have a good time. They had a ton of friends who would help out. I watched as they whispered to each other, their scheme unfolding. Marsha reached over and patted his salt and pepper beard. We tried to deem them chairs of our first fundraiser, but they just wanted to handle the raffle. Handle it they did, making the rounds at all their haunts and selling over $5,000 worth of tickets. The entire raffle raised $6,600—major money for us in those days.

Anna Belle took over the rest of the event. First, she convinced the folks at the SPJST Lodge to donate their grand ballroom and give up their normal rental charge of $500. Next, she and Dixie found three Country Western bands to donate an hour apiece of their time. So we had the place, the raffle, and the entertainment all lined up. Now all we needed was the food.

From the beginning, there was always some wonderful benefactor or two who helped cover the cost of the shrimp and somehow we managed to get everything else donated. We spent the best part of a month gathering auction items and getting commitments for food. The first year, Marsha convinced a farmer friend to deliver his donation, 400 pounds of potatoes, straight to the hall. Usually we weren't that lucky.

Daily, folks would stop at our center, bringing more stuff until there wasn't an open spot left anywhere. Volunteers canvassed local grocery stores, securing butter and cooking oil, onions and spices, tea and coffee.

For the first decade of events, Ola Mae provided the hush puppies, the bags filled up half of her freezer, and Shirley brought all the paper goods, bags of plasticware, one thousand each of dinner plates, dessert plates, paper cups and glasses, hundreds of napkins.

Jim and his friend Neil drove a huge cooking trailer over to the Lodge and set it up, sprawling out over four parking spots. Neil would pay his workers to come help move the huge pots and burners, and they all stayed outside cooking up the shrimp, potatoes, and corn on the cob.

The SPJST ballroom would reek for weeks from the smell of shrimp. There'd be a lot of fussing about it among the Lodge members, but somehow they'd forgive us and allow us to use the hall the next year.

When that first Sunday finally arrived, people were lined up around the block waiting for us to open. At eight bucks a piece it was a great deal!

The hall was too large to have a real live auction. The acoustics and sound system were great for bands, but bad for auctioneers. But we gave it a try. No one could hear, but folks would raise their hands anyway and someone would capture the prize. We've auctioned off anything and everything. Linda and Dick donated rooms full of furniture, my cousin Chris gave us one of his handmade six-foot wooden gliders, dinners at local restaurants, garden supplies, it didn't matter, if it could raise money, we wanted it.

There were two or three 'walkabouts' involving volunteers going from table to table selling chances for the fifty-fifty money pots. The Cake Walk was a hit with the kids. Throughout the day, our official money changer, Helen, would make the rounds picking up raffle money, cake money, door money, then disappear into the back room to deposit the bag of money in the Lodge's safe. Those piles of dollars would take a long time to count at the end of the day, or at least we hoped that they would.

About a third of the folks who bought tickets for the event also donated some kind of dessert. Ten tables were lined with slices of homemade cakes and pies and bags of cookies. Then the same folks would turn around and pay a dollar extra for dessert. Like I said, our fundraiser was a community affair.

Traditions get started at events like this, and one of them was that Dixie always showed up wearing the shortest shorts around. She definitely had the legs for it, and the guys loved it. She'd stand just inside the entry, serving as the official greeter.

Her patients loved talking to Dixie and Dixie loved talking to them. She often said that the best part of her job was talking to her patients. "What other work would let me spend the day getting to gossip and visit with people?" she'd say. "I love hearing about my patients, what they are doing, what's happening in their lives. It doesn't even feel like work."

I suspect her patients accounted for about half of the folks who attended. The other half was divided between folks from my church, employees, volunteers and their families, most of the operating room staff from the hospital, plus a passel of cowboys and cowgirls who went on trail rides with Dixie. Sometimes those folks came in having spent most of the previous night getting into the spirit of the day.

Looking out over the crowd was like looking into the face of The Rose. You'd see some people wearing their Sunday finest, others in jeans and cowboy hats, a bunch were in tee-shirts and shorts, and there'd be a couple of priestly collars sprinkled in. There were light faces and dark faces. A couple of clowns (the real kind) entertained with face painting and balloons. I would spot one of our sponsored women bringing in a cake and see another standing next to the local bank president behind the serving line, both intent on dishing up the shrimp.

Having volunteers around before any event is important, there's always a lot of stuff to carry over. Pam was one of the folks who offered to help. Like almost all of our employees during those early years, she started as a volunteer. Pam ended up being our chief financial officer. That first year someone gave us a mounted wild turkey, its wingspan must have been five feet from tip to tip, and the donor was convinced it was a great auction item, saying anyone would want to have it hanging on their wall! But transporting it to the Lodge required a police escort, or at least that's how it turned out. The only vehicle that was large enough to carry that thing was Pam's great white Chevy van, the kind with the bucket seats that sat seven to eight people. She put that turkey on the passenger's seat, with the top of it leaning out the window, its wing reaching out as if signaling a turn.

I admit it had to have been an odd sight with that wing and head hanging out the window, but that alone wouldn't have done it. Maybe it was the overloaded van, packed floor to ceiling with boxes, or the way the van swerved when Pam reached over to steady that turkey.

Whatever it was, something caught a policeman's eye, and next thing she knew he was pulling her over. Thank goodness he'd already bought his ticket to the Shrimp Boil or he might not have believed her story.

That first year about 600 folks showed up and most of them had an opinion about how to do it better next year. Some folks danced, others ate and visited. Over the years, there has been different entertainment, square dancers showed off one year, ballroom dancers the next, but the Country Western theme was primary.

It was several years before we discovered we could buy frozen shrimp and forgo the de-heading. It took us a few more years to figure out frozen corn on the cob was almost as good as fresh. But even without the de-heading or corn shucking, for years we continued to arrive early on Saturday night to fix the little individual cocktail sauces and set up the silent auction.

That first year was a $10,000 success, a figure that steadily grew, and by year twelve, we reached $60,000. By 2001, I had this insane idea that the event had grown stale and we needed a change. But my plan didn't work, there were too many people involved who wouldn't let the Shrimp Boil die.

When Jim retired and moved away, new people volunteered to keep it going. Mark brought a new team of cookers and Judy stepped in to corral everyone, and soon it reached a new total, raising over $100,000. Those two are still at it today.

We never would have made it through that first year without the bearded man and his sexy wife. Jim was the 'Captain' of the Shrimp Boil for ten years, later he took on more serious roles for The Rose, like serving on the board of directors.

I didn't tell Jim or Marsha about my dream. They'd understand, though. They are those special kind of people who know we don't accomplish this work alone.

Call it God or the Universe, receiving a rose from St. Theresa or finding a penny from heaven sent by Regina's mother, there seems to be some other force at work.

People often ask if we are faith based. I respond, "Hell yes we are." It takes a lot of faith to keep The Rose going.

But as great as the Shrimp Boil was, it soon became clear we were going to need a whole bunch more to keep going. We needed moneyed champions and major help.

Chapter 6
Building The Rose

Dixie rarely had the desire to go to evening meetings, especially if they were in Houston, so I was surprised when she called me all excited about going into the city to attend a Texas Executive Women's meeting. Seems she had discovered that Carolyn Farb was going to be the guest speaker, and Dixie was determined to meet this lady.

"Something tells me she could be important to The Rose," she said. All the way over to the meeting she kept affirming that we'd get to meet Carolyn and actually talk to her. Dixie believed in affirmations.

"If I can get two minutes with her," Dixie's enthusiasm was contagious, "I know I can convince her. She just needs to hear about what we are doing. She'll be excited about helping us."

This was in late 1989, and we sure needed someone to be excited about helping us. Carolyn Farb was definitely a 'bold face type,' someone whose name appears often and in bold print in the newspaper. She was a mover and shaker in the community. Any charity event listing her as the chairperson was a guaranteed success. Hers was one of the most photographed faces in Houston, featured regularly in both major newspapers and all the local rags targeting the inner circle crowds.

So we showed up at the meeting and the TEW members made a big fuss over Dixie, introducing her to the crowd as one of their first Women on the Move. It was a good start. I knew Carolyn couldn't have missed that intro or the attention that was lavished on Dixie. Besides, Dixie looked great that evening; she stood out in her red suit, and her big black and gold earrings complemented her shiny frosted hair. She exuded importance.

We were sitting in the front row as Carolyn gave her talk. It was a good one, full of dos and don'ts for fundraising. Carolyn's style and delivery was pure confidence. She seldom smiled and referred to her notes often. When she did make eye contact it was deliberate and focused. Her words were concise and to the point. Her gleaming white designer suit wrapped perfectly around her slender body and set off her long blond hair.

When she finished and the meeting was officially closed, folks continued to mingle. Dixie was primed. We waited until the waters of people parted from around Carolyn. I gave Dixie a little push. Suddenly she was face to face with her, towering over Carolyn, the high heels making her even taller. It's difficult to ignore Dixie anytime, but next to impossible when she wears red.

I held my breath, watching as she launched into her spiel. Carolyn stared at her wide-eyed.

"Hi, I'm Dixie Melillo and that was a wonderful speech. Everything you said about raising money is exactly what we needed to hear. We've started The Rose, Dorothy and I," she motioned at me, "It's a non-profit and we're providing free mammograms to women who don't have insurance. You cannot imagine how many women there are who need help. Breast cancer is a big issue and women can't afford mammograms." Dixie never took a breath and continued talking nonstop for at least two minutes, ending it with, "We sure could use your help. We just need some guidance about what we should do next."

At that point, Carolyn moved her head, looked at her, then turned and walked away. She never acknowledged Dixie, never said a word or changed the expression on her face. It was as though Carolyn hadn't seen her. In fact, I don't remember her blinking the entire time Dixie was talking.

Dixie stood there with her mouth open. I was equally shocked. Several of the women were starting to gather around us, wanting to catch a quick visit with the doctor and tease her about being a wayward member. Dixie's eyes followed Carolyn's retreating figure as it walked through the crowd and left the room. She regained her composure and became her usual friendly self.

Before long we were making our way down the road for that long journey back to her office in Pasadena. It was late, we were tired, and we didn't talk much. That was an oddity for us.

Two years later, Dixie got a call at her office.

"Dixie," the voice had a cultured quality to it, there was no mistaking it. "I've been thinking about what we were talking about, and I want you to meet the Cancer Fighters. They've received a special bequest from a member's estate and I think there could be an interest in The Rose." Carolyn paused before saying, "I don't have time to talk now. I wanted to give you a quick call and see if you'd check your calendar. When would be a good time for you? I want to set up a meeting between you and their president."

Of course, Dixie never knew that I had sent a proposal to Carolyn. But still, that had been after that fateful conversation at the TEW meeting. I was as surprised as Dixie over the call.

So began our 'on again, off again' relationship with Carolyn. It would span the next decade and include a dozen different types of encounters. One of the first calls she made when she was diagnosed with breast cancer was to Dixie.

We suspected there was a special way of doing things among the rich and famous, and that we'd probably never totally figure it out. We learned early on that the Universe seems to have its own time schedule.

During those years, Dixie and I kept reminding each other that some things aren't meant to be and we had to be patient. Fortunately, meeting with the Cancer Fighters was one of those 'meant to be things,' and we soon discovered that our time of being around the rich and famous had just begun.

True to her word, Carolyn arranged a meeting with the key folks of the Cancer Fighters. Five of the most polished, well dressed, and wealthiest women that I'd ever met sat on our donated chairs in the tiny reception area of The Rose, discussing our future and their goals. Butterflies filled my stomach as I tried to sit still in that circle of women.

"Yes, we would be interested in helping set up a second center for The Rose, one located inside the 610 loop."

Listening to the women talk was like being in a dream—one that was about to come true. Carolyn, Dr. Jane, Alysse, Ann, and Linda made up the search committee for the next project of the Cancer Fighters. One of their charter members, Joan Gordon, had died and left $10,000 in her will for a service project that was meaningful. A few weeks later, they met with their membership and soon we were notified. Their new 'service' project would become The Rose Joan Gordon Center.

This was 1990, and I knew that $10,000 would barely cover opening a place, much less running it. I sure didn't want to discourage them, but I'd learned my lesson of scrimping by for so many years and never having quite enough funding to move forward. Their answer was to host an elaborate fundraiser at the River Oaks home of the Mecoms. Susie Taylor, a breast cancer survivor and a Cancer Fighter, spearheaded the event, and to this day I don't think there has ever been an evening as elegant or graceful as that one.

Driving up the winding pathway to the palatial estate on Lazy Lane and seeing the River Oaks mansion for the first time was a once in a lifetime event. Larger than life bronze statues of bulls and other animals framed the oversized driveway, and the fountains, gardens, and long hanging boughs of ancient hundred-year-old oak trees created an 'other worldly' entrance. Somewhere on the grounds was a sunken tennis court, man-made lakes, a guest house, and a putting green. We never saw any of the grounds, wandering around the first level of the 14,000 square foot mansion was more than enough, and nothing was more impressive than the majestic staircase and entrance. Each room was museum perfect and became another adventure in seeing the world through the hundreds of antiques and rare collections gathered by the two generations of Mecoms.

Oil millionaire, owner of the New Orleans Saints and more, John Mecom, Jr. and his mother, grand matriarch Mary, were the most gracious of hosts. His wife Katsy had recently finished her own ordeal with breast cancer, and she and Dixie immediately hit it off.

The evening raised $25,000, and with Joan's original $10,000, we were off and running. By April, 1991, an empty shell of space in a strip shopping center had carpet, drapes, chairs, medical equipment, office furnishings, and supplies. The Rose Joan Gordon Center was opened.

One of the reasons this place was so attractive to us was its reasonable rent. I soon learned that this location was cheap for two reasons. One was the actual location, it was at the very end of a strip center that dead ended into a fence and had an alley that ran behind it. I wasn't worried that the place had bars across the windows or on its one door. But during that first year I became intimately aware of the reasons they were there.

One Monday morning, around 8:30, I drove up to the center. My mind was totally focused on starting the day. The moment I opened the car door, I was dragged out by a guy holding a knife and demanding my purse as he pulled it off my shoulder and pushed me to the ground. I never saw the car drive up behind him and was only vaguely aware of him getting into it. The bounce on the concrete was hard enough to bruise my head pretty badly. But other than peeing all over myself when he first dragged me out, and being totally shaken, I was okay. Actually, it would be months before I was really okay, but at least I was alive and unhurt.

I stumbled inside, locked the door behind me, and tried to think. I didn't know what to do. I called the police, who after grudgingly recording the incident, advised me these kinds of events were a regular happening in that neighborhood and I needed to "be more careful."

More careful? I was incensed! My thoughts leapt to the next evening, when our support group would be meeting. Women battling for their lives, women tired and depleted from chemotherapy. What if those men returned and attacked them? I remember standing at the receptionist counter, trembling, looking out past those black bars that covered the windows. What if they came back now? My heart started to pound and fear walked into the room.

Finally the two staff folks arrived, and minutes later the volunteers; soon patients would be coming for their appointments. My words were matter of fact and my voice was calm as I told my staff that I had been robbed and I needed to go home to change clothes. I cautioned them to be extra careful. By the time I reached home and pushed open the door the phone was ringing. Anna Belle's voice shouted at me over the phone lines. She demanded details and was furious that I had not called. I had no business driving, she lectured, no business even thinking about returning to work.

Later in the week the police did come to the center and I identified one of the men from a photo library, but I wasn't sure about the other one, the one who had driven the black El Camino, I had only gotten a glimpse of him. That was too bad, they said, they needed confirmation on both men, but they admitted they knew those guys, both had a record of robberies and assaults.

Traumas of violence mess with our minds. I became incredibly paranoid. I couldn't stop thinking that those two men knew where I lived. We rekeyed the house but I still didn't feel safe. I checked and rechecked the locks, added gates to the car port, and many nights I woke up imagining someone had found a way in.

The other change I made was to install a magnetic door so we could control who entered the Center. One of the service folks brought me a small gun. I hate to admit it now, but I actually took it. We kept it hidden in the tech area. We also installed a blue alarm light that was controlled by the front desk person. It would flash in the tech area if the front desk person was in trouble. The tech was supposed to call 911 when it started flashing, which of course it did more than once—always by accident when a volunteer leaned against it. It wasn't long before the tech learned to call the front desk before calling 911.

The second reason that center's rent was so cheap was that it was located next to a pet store, which had a chronic unpleasant odor that permeated into our space, and a problem of escaping animals, mainly white rats, that always made it to our side of the building.

But somehow we managed. Our furnishings were nice enough, our equipment was good, our techs were great, and we had a host of volunteers to help with the day-to-day.

There were three volunteers in particular who came on a regular basis. Linda was one of them, not only was she president of the Cancer Fighters and a champion fundraiser, but she also spent hours each week covering our telephone and being our receptionist.

One day, I was in the back, sitting at my donated, falling apart desk located behind a partition, while Linda was covering the front reception area, standing behind a tall counter concocted from the remnants of someone's showroom. I heard the door buzzer and the familiar click of the release of the magnetic strip that allowed our patients to enter.

A young mother came through the door with her two children and settled them in the reception area. Linda later told me that that young woman had such a concerned look on her face when she came up to the counter, Linda knew she was really upset and totally stressed out. The woman whispered to Linda that several months ago she had found a lump in her breast. She explained that she didn't have much money so she had had to wait to see a doctor. Someone told her about The Rose.

I could almost hear their conversation; the place was so small voices traveled easily over and around the temporary partitions and file cabinets. But I wasn't really paying attention until I realized Linda's voice was becoming louder and louder.

"He told you what?" I heard her say sharply. "He told you to watch your lump and come back in six months? Let me tell you one thing, if your doctor had a lump on his penis you can be sure that he would not 'watch it' for six months!"

I screeched and jumped out of my chair, heading to the front. I couldn't believe my ears. What on earth was she saying to a patient?

To this day, Linda still laughs at my reaction, she was fearless and undeterred when it came to speaking her mind about what women should know and do. She also reminds me that I promptly moved her to the back office area where she tried to hold her tongue 'in check.'

"But you relented, Dorothy. After a while you let me go back to the front desk," she would giggle and add, "You <u>had</u> to! I was the only help you had on some days."

And she was right. But saying that I would actually 'screech' at volunteers was an exaggeration. Well, sometimes it was. Sometimes it was the only option I had. Overseeing this team of volunteers was a feat in itself. These were strong women, used to doing things their way.

Another screech came the day I heard Suzanne, one of the regular volunteers, giving instructions to a patient over the telephone. She had finished gathering all the personal information, name, date of birth, referring doctor, and giving her directions to the center, when I heard her say, "Be sure to wear a two piece outfit and don't put on any deodorant." There was a pause, and then I heard her say, "Oh, that's okay. If you forget about the deodorant, we'll just take you outside and hose you down!"

I screeched big time at that one, only to learn she was talking to a friend. While she dissolved into laughter, I dissolved into relief.

But it was Zoraida, our one and only Spanish-speaking volunteer, who stole my heart while bringing her own unique challenge. One look at this tiny, gorgeous knockout of a Venezuelan woman and you knew she was in a league all her own. She spoke with a rich, thick accent and her sentences were equally rich with adjectives. Her voice was alive with excitement and filled with laughter. Listening to her translations with patients and hoping she was saying exactly what I had told her to say was a minor problem. The real challenge was that she wore the most incredibly revealing, shortest skirts and lowest cleavage exposing tops. In fact, hers were the sexiest clothes ever seen on a woman in public, at least in our public.

"Remember, Zoraida," I lectured as I reached for her top and tried in vain to pull it up an inch more, "We are a breast cancer center. You can't go around showing off your breasts like that!"

"I don't understand, Do-ro-thee," her rich accent stretched out each syllable of my name as she rolled the 'r.' She looked down at her chest then stared up at me, and said innocently, "These are my breasts. They are there and the clothes fit around them. I don't understand what you mean showing-off?"

After a while, I gave up, to heck with my fuddy-duddy worries about professional appearance. She worked magic with our Spanish-speaking patients and that was all that mattered.

There were so many other volunteers who kept us going, I wish I could name them all. The Cancer Fighters continue to be part of our life.

One of the happiest days in my life was when we moved out of that location on Stella Link and said goodbye to the run-down shopping center, the bars on the windows, and runaway mice. We had suffered through five long years and the day after our lease was up we were out of there. By then, I had hired Amy, and we had enough patients to actually be a viable center.

When we moved from that space, Amy called me and said, "What do you want me to do with the G.U.N?"

We always spelled out the word, as if doing that made having one more acceptable.

"Oh, take it with you and I'll pick it up tomorrow," I responded, not thinking.

So Amy set off with it, her van piled high with boxes, driving through the city with a concealed weapon hidden under her seat! The next day I relieved her of gun control duty.

"What were we thinking?" Amy and I ask each other now.

"Having a gun in the center?" But we did a lot of things then that we would never dream of doing now.

It was summer of 1996 when we moved into a wonderful new space in a modern medical building located on Bissonnet, in a section of town that was nice. We had a prime first floor location in a building that was secure and well kept. We were so excited to be in a space that we could be proud of, and even more excited about having space to add ultrasound services and still have lots of room to grow.

We were on our way.

Chapter 7
The Tech from Texas

There are some people you know you're going to like even before you meet them, and Amy was one of them. Everything on her resume was perfect: she was a registered mammography technologist and she had run a busy mammogram center for a dozen plus years. Her experience and credentials were flawless, and to top it off her middle name was Rose. That had to be a good omen. The only problem was she lived in Longview (about four hours north of Houston) and she wouldn't be available for work for two months.

Amy will tell you I hired her on the spot during that first telephone interview, and that's pretty much true. She was responding to an ad in the paper and had called for information. I basically offered her the job, sight unseen. She was flabbergasted and didn't accept until she received my offer letter and saw the return address and the words: "The Rose."

She told her fiancé that she was going to work for us. When he figured out where The Rose Joan Gordon Center was located, he tried to reason with her. "Are you out of your mind? Do you have any idea how far you'll drive every day? There are three hospitals between our home and that place! You could go to work at any one of them!"

From the sound of her voice and the way she spoke, I fully expected to meet a petite blond who was young and maybe just a wee bit of an airhead. While Amy did turn out to be small (weren't we all back then?), she was the same age as me, and her black hair and bushy eyebrows that nearly met in the middle of her face destroyed my blond theory. The idea of her being an airhead was also pretty much expelled, except for the fact that she did talk a lot. She still does. Amy can talk about anything and everything and for extended amounts of time. When she is on a roll, she seldom comes up for air. When she is quiet, someone is in trouble. Her ability to talk has gotten us out of some type of jam more than once, and gotten us into a lot of crazy adventures.

Amy handled our first accreditation. That was a major deal back then, it still is today. But 1992 was a time when mammogram centers had just started being accredited and there were lots of questions about the process and the required documentation.

The state inspector came after the physicist had done his or her survey, which was another whole process and usually involved corrections on the machines. Our machines were pretty sound, and the corrections were never anything major but always a hassle.

The first time I went through an inspection with Amy, we had worked till 3 o'clock in the morning reviewing and readying our paperwork. We had met at her house and spread everything out over her dining room table. She was very methodical and checked and rechecked everything several times. We had hauled over one of those huge old pre-computer IBM typewriters, just in case we found anything that needed to be retyped in our procedures. We compared the regulations line by line against our process, ensuring everything the regulations required was written down and consistent with what we did. We filled up two three-inch, three-ring binders and still had a box full of other paperwork. I left her house feeling like things were pretty much in order.

I didn't personally witness what happened that next day but it was verified by more than one person, some of whom were looking out the window while eating breakfast at Alfred's, the restaurant located across from our center. The story has also made the rounds among the tales told by state workers, ultimately labeled as the most unbelievable inspection in the history of mammography. And of course, the inspector has his own version.

It seems that Amy was running a little late that morning. The inspector had already arrived. He had parked a little ways down from the front of the center, under the one shade tree, and was sitting in his car, just waiting, minding his own business. The noise behind him made him check his rearview mirror as a huge blue van filled up his vision. It was turning a bit too sharply and appeared to be balancing on two wheels. He held his breath, thinking it was coming straight at him, when it careened back around and narrowly missed the bumper of his car.

No one ever parks there! Amy sniffed to herself, not suspecting the car's ownership. She screeched to a stop, bumping the front end of the van against the curb, making its big old body bounce back and forth. She opened the van's door and jumped out, immediately slamming herself up against the running board and back into the van as she tried to simultaneously toss two huge bags over her shoulder.

Recovered, with bags in place, she turned, facing the van, and started pulling at something that was behind the driver's seat. A few more tugs and an old black purse, almost as big as the bags, popped out at her, spewing items all over the sidewalk.

Growling, she bent over, snatched them up one by one and stuffed them back into the purse. Then she started digging in that same monster-sized purse. A few moments passed, then she smacked one hand against her forehead, the keys she was searching for dangled from her other hand.

At that point, she started walking toward the front door of the center.

The inspector had watched her arrival and decided to give her a few minutes to open up. When he started to get out of his car, he realized she had come back outside. He stopped and waited and watched.

Amy vanished around the side of the van and he could barely see her opening the sliding doors through the windows of the van. Then she walked back into the center carrying the three-ring binders atop a big box.

Two seconds later, she was back outside, and again went around to the side of the van. When she came back into view this time she was balancing a laundry basket against one hip, it was stacked with folded cover-ups, and she had a full to overflowing bag of groceries on the other hip. (Our washer had been on the blink, so she had carried the towels home to launder, and it was support group night, hence the goodies.)

On the fourth trip, she was loaded down with hangers of clothes and two shoe boxes, another trip in and out.

The fifth time she emerged from the side of the van, she was bent over, holding the old IBM typewriter close against her stomach. She sort of struggled forward, shuffling a bit, and nearly tripped on the curb. The inspector was out of his car, moving toward her, ready to help, but she had propped open the front door of the center and was inside before he had rounded the back end of his car.

Actually, he had become a bit mesmerized by this back and forth parade, or so he told folks later.

What happened next was straight out of a bad vaudeville act. Amy returned and walked directly to the back of the van. She opened the doors, reached into the van and pulled out an ironing board. Yes, an ironing board.

At the very moment the board cleared the van, the legs sprang open with a loud pop. She stumbled backwards, almost falling into the inspector.

When he said, "Can I help you?" she screamed and swung around, seeing him for the first time. Of course, she was still holding that ironing board, so when she swung around its legs were poking straight ahead and grazed the inspector.

Amy was mortified and started talking. There was a function that day, she explained, with the Cancer Fighters. She went on to tell him who the Cancer Fighters were, how they had started the second center, how we really needed the money and how she had to go to this function. She had brought a different outfit to wear that needed to be touched up. The function wasn't until 4 p.m., but with the inspection, she wouldn't have time to go home.

She rattled on and on, peering out from behind the ironing board. Then she spied his arm and started apologizing. He stood there, first staring at her and then at the blood trickling down to his wrist.

When he finally did go inside, she kept asking him if he was really hurt and insisted on doctoring the scratches. She tried her best to make him feel better by bringing him snacks in between each set of paperwork. It was going to be a long three days.

It stands to reason that no one would purposely manhandle a state inspector. One failing grade and the center would be closed. Actually, the inspector took a lot of smoke breaks that day. Pity, since he said he'd almost beat that habit. Amy said he seemed a bit nervous, but then who wouldn't be after being attacked by an ironing board?

The next day, he arrived at the main office and things went from bad to worse. In the middle of inspecting the second of two machines, its light field didn't work right. Over the years, the light field had been a minor but persistent problem on this machine. It had been corrected time and again by the service guys. In fact, it had been fixed the week before and had been in perfect alignment, but not on this day.

This kind of problem would mean it wouldn't pass. It wasn't a serious violation, but it would have been a ding on Amy's record. Something she would not allow.

Amy barged into my office, her face flushed, those dark eyebrows knotted together. She slammed her fists on my desk, leaned forward, and in a voice a little too loud, said, "Remember we talked about replacing Unit 2?"

I nodded.

"Well, today's the day we get rid of it!"

"What? Wait a minute, Amy. What do you mean? We haven't raised the money for a new one. We can't just get rid of this one."

"Oh yes we can!" she emphasized each word, her eyes flashing. "I've already called Ron and he's sending his guys over to move it out."

"What?"

"It won't pass. That stupid light field again. So I asked the inspector, 'What would happen if it weren't here?' He said he couldn't inspect what wasn't there. So I unplugged it and it's out of here…TODAY!"

I sighed. There was never any arguing with Amy once her mind was made up.

When the three days of inspection finally came to an end, the three of us, Amy, the inspector and I, gathered in my office. Amy and I sat on one side of my desk, she in a chair pulled close to the corner, and the inspector sat on the other side. He spread out paperwork, made faces, and tapped a sheet here or there before starting the debriefing. We held our breath. He looked up and began a long drawn out explanation of what he had inspected, what the parameters were, why they were important, and how difficult it was for any mammography center to pass inspection on the first round.

In the end, the only words we heard were, "You passed!"

Simultaneously, Amy and I burst out crying and started hugging each other (in our usual professional manner)! The inspector, Ray, just shook his head.

Many years later, Amy heard that Ray was terminally ill, lung cancer. In her normal way, she reached out to him, sending a note, telling him we had added him to our prayer list. He responded, thanking her for her kind words and teasing her about that first visit. Just like Amy herself, he remarked, "It was unforgettable."

In all the years to follow, we always had 100% perfect inspections. Not a small feat, but only one of many on Amy's list of accomplishments. It was Amy who convinced, Lazlo Tabar, MD, the radiologist who set the gold standards for film mammography and the most famous mammographer in the world, to visit our center. It was Amy who convinced Ward Parsons, MD, an equally famous physician, to come to work for us. It was Amy who initiated the most successful—by number of attendees and years running— mammography technologist seminars in Houston. For years they were sold out months before the date of the event. It was Amy who initiated one of the first 3-D ultrasound programs in the nation and made The Rose the fifth center in Texas to offer an advanced nuclear medicine program for the breast.

Perhaps her greatest legacy was launching our mobile mammography program in 2006. It was another first in Texas and those units didn't require the million dollar oversized coaches that took half a dozen parking spaces. Instead, her program used small vans to transport the portable mammography equipment to the site. Those mammography machines literally rolled inside buildings, set up in any ten by ten foot room, and were ready for business within minutes.

Soon we had a fleet of vans and corporate clients as well as community clinics booking the units a year in advance. That program alone was responsible for The Rose receiving multi-million dollar grants that allowed us to serve most of rural Texas. The concept was novel, it was cost effective, it made sense, and it was Amy whose work and dedication made it happen.

Not bad for a tech from Texas.

Chapter 8
Women of Class

The first time I met Nancy Brinker, founder of Susan G. Komen for the Cure, I was standing in the middle of Tiffany's in the Galleria, attending a 'by invitation only' event along with a crowd of about eighty of Houston's elite and socially significant. The gleaming glass counters and shelves were filled with thousands of dollars worth of diamonds and crystal. As we juggled tiny cups of coffee and plates of sweets, Dixie joked about not making any sudden moves. "This is the real stuff," she teased.

It was a morning coffee to kick off the Race for the Cure, the 5K Walk/Run that was sponsored by the Houston affiliate of The Susan G. Komen Breast Cancer Foundation. The Houston affiliate was just over a year old but they had already awarded The Rose a $9,000 grant, the second largest grant we had ever received. It was 9:30 a.m., and if things didn't get started soon we were going to have to leave—patients would be waiting. Suddenly there was a commotion near the entrance, and a tall, stately woman emerged through the crowd.

Hundreds of stories have been written about Nancy Brinker and her promise to younger sister Susan, who was dying of breast cancer. It was a promise that led to the creation of an organization that would soon span the nation and raise millions of dollars for breast cancer screening, education, and research.

As many times as I had seen pictures of Nancy, nothing prepared me for her dynamic presence. She was tall, maybe five foot eight or more. Her chin length, thick jet black hair was pulled back behind her ears. It bounced slightly as she walked. A pair of big black-framed glasses set off her strong, square attractive face. The black hair and black glasses against her pale skin gave her a signature look that was even more accentuated by her broad shoulders. She had the unmistakable look of the wealthy, and she moved with a sense of power.

She completed her ten minute rah-rah speech, and then someone acknowledged Dr. Melillo and asked her to say a few words about The Rose. Dixie kept it short and appreciative. At the end of it, someone from the crowd tossed out what seemed to be an innocent question.

"But, don't you charge some women for a mammogram?"

Dixie answered yes, saying any woman could come to us for a mammogram. She proudly noted that our $50 fee, which included the radiologist's charges, was certainly less than anywhere else in town. Then she added, "At $50, we don't even cover our costs."

That same person replied, "Then maybe we shouldn't be going to The Rose if doing a mammogram is costing you money."

I jumped in and started to explain how important that revenue was in giving us the base for our work.

The woman interrupted, "I was at The Rose the other day and there was not one Race for the Cure brochure anywhere, not in the lobby or in the exam rooms."

I felt like a bucket of cold water had been thrown on me. I was so embarrassed. She was right; we didn't have any brochures at either center. I hadn't thought about it and didn't even know where to get them.

I was mentally beating myself up when Nancy interceded and said, "What this sounds like to me is an excellent volunteer opportunity." And in the next moment she had two members recruited to deliver a box of race brochures to each center by that afternoon. That's class.

Since then, the Houston affiliate has been one of our greatest supporters. I am absolutely clear that The Rose would not exist today were it not for their generosity and belief in us. Not a year has passed that their funding didn't fill a critical need or catapult us into new arenas of service.

First they funded mammograms. When we needed diagnostic capabilities, they paved the way, providing support for ultrasound systems and funding the entire stereotactic biopsy suite. These systems represented nearly a million dollars worth of equipment; they were top of the line and state of the art. The Houston affiliate's commitment to us meant our patients, rich or poor, insured or not, received an uncompromised level of service.

That voice from the crowd may not have been one of our fans, but she sure was an excellent teacher. We never missed a chance in the future to promote the race or be a part of their events.

The curious thing about The Rose was that, despite all the good work or all the women we cared for, we couldn't quite capture the attention (which translates into financial commitment) from the local rich and famous. People would see articles in the paper about them and immediately call me, rattling away, "All you need to do is get in touch with so and so. They have lots of money. Just ask them for a donation, look at what they just gave the Medical Center…or Baylor College of Medicine…or MD Anderson."

Of course, those same people, well-intentioned all, didn't personally know "so and so," didn't have a clue how to contact them, and didn't understand that having "lots of money" isn't always the primary factor in a donation.

Sometimes we'd hear, second or third hand, that some prominent person thought The Rose was a wonderful story and our work with those poor people was commendable, but our mission just didn't tug at their hearts or we didn't have enough 'curb appeal.' I guess there is some truth to that thinking. There's not much that is glamorous about diagnosing breast cancer or about being poor and needing health services, especially when living in the shadow of the largest medical center in the nation.

We were told that we "didn't have any big names" on our board of directors. That criticism always chapped me. Our board moved The Rose from nothing to a major healthcare player in the city, big names or not. But the mantra of the non-profit world of "Who's on your board?" isn't a question; it's a statement of perceived status.

I'd attended enough non-profit events to know the importance of success stories. What audience wouldn't respond to hearing the story of a battered woman who fled in the middle of the night with nothing but her children and who is now CEO of a local business? Or what about the before and after graphics showing the transformation of a poorly dressed single mom who's gone to school at night to get her certification and finally landed the job of her dreams after being dressed 'correctly' for the interview? Who wouldn't be touched by the images of helpless puppies and kittens about to be put to death because they hadn't been adopted?

Our compelling stories involved women who didn't have insurance and our service was in diagnosing the disease, not treating it. It took me a while to realize that there's a lot of inherent prejudice towards the uninsured. They're often characterized as lazy indigents who won't work for a living or who are illegal aliens. Truth of the matter is most of our sponsored women work hard to make a living. They work at low paying jobs, the ones that don't offer group health insurance. A small percentage of our sponsored women have been laid off or have gone through some other life changing event that meant losing their insurance coverage—such as divorce.

One of the saddest cases was the 63-year-old whose husband had left her for a younger woman and taken the insurance coverage with him. It was all she could do to find any kind of work at that age, and she was banking on staying healthy until she was 65 and eligible for Medicare. The lump in her breast put a crimp in that idea. Did we ultimately help her get coverage through Social Security Medicaid/Medicare? Yes. It took months of processing paperwork, but we got it. Did she get treatment? Yes. Did she ever reclaim her dignity? No.

I could sometimes get through to the unbelieving by asking them what would happen if they lost their job and insurance. How long could they afford to pay an average of $1,000 a month for Cobra coverage, especially if there wasn't any money coming in? How long would they take the chance on going without insurance? What if they thought there was another job right around the corner? Would they chance having no insurance for one month? Three?

At that stage in our existence, I had gathered over a hundred cases of women finding a lump in their breast during the first three months without insurance coverage.

Telling our story also meant fighting the prevailing misconception that the poor could access healthcare anytime they wanted, either through the County Hospital Districts or, if they had cancer, MD Anderson. Anyone could get into the public health system at Ben Taub Hospital, that's a true statement, but the cost of services was dictated by a person's income. If you happened to be totally indigent, you were eligible for free services. Heaven forbid that a person attempt to stay off the public dole and try to earn a living. It was the ultimate irony that totally indigent women received the full range of care, from mastectomy to chemotherapy to radiation therapy to reconstruction, all free of charge, while the working poor got only what they could afford.

No insurance and get into MD Anderson without money? Not likely, especially if you made more than $3,000 a year and lived in Houston. According to the state, Ben Taub was the approved facility for residents of Harris County. Oh, it's true the occasional uninsured patient would get into a clinical trial at MD Anderson, but she had to have one of the wild types of cancer.

The maze of rules and regulations grew more complex and the changing criteria for eligibility were maddening.

Dixie had referred one woman to UTMB in Galveston for her mastectomy and chemotherapy treatments. Dixie knew about Pat's financial struggle. She and her husband operated a small plant nursery that could barely eke out a living. Unfortunately, the profits were gobbled up by the medication expenses needed for her recently diagnosed diabetic husband.

Any hopes of finding another job were squelched when she weighed it against the time involved in caring for the special needs of their bed-ridden handicapped child. On paper, however, hers appeared to be a very different story. The business showed a profit for two out of the three years in the information she submitted when applying for public health. That and the fact that she was buying a home put her in the 100% payment range for services.

Pat carried her referral paper to UTMB, finished the approval process, and went into the hospital for her mastectomy. Before she knew it, she received her first bill for $5,000. Then she was told that chemotherapy was going to cost $400 every three weeks. She'd already signed an agreement with the hospital to pay against her account, which grew larger with each lab test or follow-up consultation. But before they would schedule her appointments for the chemotherapy, she was going to have to come up with the money up front.

When Dixie received one of those form letters sent to referring physicians advising her that her patient was non-compliant and had not returned for treatments, she immediately called Pat. Listening to Pat's story was disheartening. She was more than a little angry about the whole set up and she had no intention of going back. It wasn't just the money, but the hours and hours of waiting at the clinics that were taking a toll. She had to pay for someone to stay with her child every time she went, and often her appointments would be rescheduled or take all day.

The time she had been hospitalized had really hurt what was left of the business. She simply didn't have the money and was fighting to keep food in the house. To top things off, her husband had had a heart attack during this time and couldn't help. The hospital suggested she get a second mortgage, she couldn't have gotten one if she'd wanted to. We learned that it was common practice for hospitals to strongly 'encourage' (read 'insist') that folks remortgage their homes. For a patient who is terrified for her life, it can seem like the only solution.

Pat had decided she would just have to take her chances; hope the mastectomy got all of the cancer and do without the chemotherapy. Dixie tried to convince her otherwise, offering to call the hospital and try for new arrangements. Dixie knew Pat really needed the chemotherapy and asked her if she understood how important the treatments were.

Pat's parting words hung in the air. "Dr. Melillo, don't you understand?" she retorted sharply, "If I'd had an extra $400 a month to shell out, I would have had insurance."

Even with our success in conveying the plight of our sponsored women to local foundations, it was a struggle to attract people of means. It was rare to find us running among the rich and famous, so those few times we did have that chance were always memorable. I could tell you the month, the time of day, and exactly what I was doing when I was introduced to one of the first rich and famous to come into our lives.

On a sunny day in October, I was sitting in Felicia's office; she was my medical records coordinator and an ace of an employee. We were working on patient reports, and knowing we were two days behind made me determined that nothing was going to distract us.

That was the moment the call from Linda Hofheinz was put through.

Hofheinz is a name that most long-term Houstonians would recognize. It was synonymous with the building of the Astrodome and linked to the infamous penthouse stories from those early days of the "eighth wonder of the world." It was the ink that formed much of the city's colorful and powerfully political mayoral history.

I cradled the telephone between my neck and ear, intent on my task, trying to do two things at once, when my pen stopped in mid-air.

The voice on the line had responded to my hello with, "I'm Linda Hofheinz and I was diagnosed with breast cancer in April of this year." Linda's voice was measured and smooth, it had an almost singsong quality to it. She articulated each word as she spoke, and her presence on the other end of the line actually filled up the space between us.

"I've been talking to Mary from the Rosebuds support group. Do you know her?" she asked. I said yes of course I did, adding that Mary had been a real supporter.

Linda continued with, "I know. Mary was telling me about The Rose. Actually, she was raving about your programs. She's a true fan of The Rose. She told me that you help women who don't have insurance or money to get mammograms. Is that correct?"

Again I said yes. My mind was going through its usual processing, trying to guess what had prompted this call.

"As I was saying, I was diagnosed in April, and I cannot imagine what it would be like to go through breast cancer without insurance or money. I have a strong support network, my husband and family have been wonderful, and I have insurance." There was a little rise in her voice, punctuating the end of her sentence.

I think I came back with some feeble response about how important it was to have support and I started to launch into all the different services we offered for uninsured women.

She stopped my dialogue by saying that Mary was very knowledgeable about our programs and how impressed she was with what Mary had shared. Then, without skipping a beat, she said, "I want to make a donation and just need to know your address. Where you would like me to send this check?"

Never in our history had anyone ever called and asked for the address to send a check. Usually I was calling people asking if I could send them information about The Rose, hoping against hope that they would read it and maybe someday be moved to indeed send a check.

I was stunned. For the briefest moment I couldn't recall the address, the silence seemed endless before I finally regrouped and stuttered through it.

She then asked if we were a 501(c)3.

I said yes, and thought I must have misunderstood what she said earlier. *She is calling for information,* I said to myself. Once I sent it to her, there would probably be some kind of long approval process.

"Would you like me to send you a proposal outlining our programs or a brochure?" I asked, my confidence returning. Proposals I knew how to do, fielding these kinds of calls I didn't. "I can get right on it," I assured her.

"No," she said sweetly, "I'm just making a note on my check." With that, she thanked me profusely for taking her call, again complimented The Rose, and with the decisiveness of a queen graciously dismissing members of her court, she gently said she really must be going and hung up.

I sat staring at the receiver in my hand until Felicia's voice pulled me back into the room.

Over the next few days, I replayed the conversation a zillion times, questioning if I had heard her correctly, wondering if I had handled the call properly. I had to chuckle when it dawned on me how easily she had stopped my dissertation about The Rose and moved the conversation to exactly where she wanted it to go. Interrupting somebody without them knowing it, and more importantly, without them caring, was a real skill.

I would soon learn that this was a woman of many skills, much diplomacy, and a steeled graciousness that made things happen. Her check in the amount of $5,000 arrived four days later. It was the largest donation from an individual that we'd ever received. It marked a turning point in our history.

Over the next few months, the calls from Linda were highlights of my day. She always had another idea that would in some way enhance our image, such as orchestrating a professionally produced brochure. The final product, an eight by twelve inch booklet, was a far cry from the three-fold single-page brochure we used. Linda convinced her friend and colleague, Steve Stanley, a top notch designer, to produce it. The look was stunning.

The story inside was written by Linda's sister, Diana Hickerson, a professional writer whose awards were equally impressive and whose writing was brilliant. Diana told our story as it had never been told before. She captured the essence of our mission and filled twelve pages with intriguing stories and an invitation to support us. She coined the phrase on its cover: "The cost of breast cancer is too high. We've made it our mission to lower it."

Next, Linda tackled our logo. "Dorothy, The Rose is not a rose," she announced. "It's not a flower, isn't that correct? Didn't you name it that because of the women who were involved in the beginning?" She added, "I've been thinking about the image of The Rose and I think I might be able to design something that would project more of what you really stand for."

She understood the importance of symbolism and created a strong logo that we would use for over a decade.

Linda would continue to weave in and out of our lives, and her presence brought moments of sunshine during a very dark and sad time in the personal life of The Rose.

Anna Belle had a reoccurrence and this cancer was especially vicious. It appeared on her annual mammogram, she hadn't been having any problems, it was a routine exam. When the tech called and said I needed to go to the mammography work area, I knew something was wrong. I pushed open the doors to see Anna Belle leaning against the wall, staring at the films on the light box. The look on her face stopped my heart. I glanced at the films; the white splotch of cancer was obvious.

"This makes me so damn mad," she said with more pure hatred than I had ever heard in anyone's voice before.

The months that followed were impossible. Anna Belle was the office manager of the main center. She held the entire operation together. Hers was the back that carried the load, and her load was about to become even heavier.

Her medical process started: biopsy, surgery, bilateral mastectomies, reconstruction, complications and chemotherapy. This time she did lose her hair, she was incredibly ill. Yet she kept on working. Through the next year and a half she maintained, trying to keep her regular schedule. But the treatment was tough and she had to move to part time.

My most cherished memories of her revolve around those last months. She'd walk into my office wearing a sassy hat or bright scarf, makeup always perfect, lipstick in place. The most important thing she wore was her 'I can beat this' face.

She might have too, if her husband of over 29 years hadn't

contracted a cancer of his own. The tumor that appeared on his arm seemed to multiply overnight, covering his body. It was leukemia, even more aggressive than what she was fighting. There were days and days of hospitalization, and countless hopes dashed as each treatment failed, and within ten months he was dead.

These two people were always together. She once told me he had no choice but to leave, he couldn't bear to see her so ill. Once he died, Anna Belle's cancer metastasized to her lungs. The battle was drawing to an end, and one day in June, she was gone.

That same two-year period marked a huge growth cycle at The Rose. The Rose Joan Gordon Center was bulging at its seams and months were spent finding it a larger, new home.

We opened The Rose on Vista in Pasadena, which immediately became incredibly busy and was a huge success. A year later, we opened a small screening center across town, which proved to be a short-lived disaster.

We jumped from seven employees to twenty-one employees and had to lease extra office space for the main center. New funding meant computerizing our system and attempting to combine our different data bases, a feat we never quite achieved. We were involved in more fundraisers than ever before and received publicity that would have made major corporations envious.

Linda's intuition about The Rose needing a new image was on target. We were leaving behind an old way of being and entering into a new one. We had no option, the number of women needing our help exploded, forcing us into new areas and levels of service.

As much as I welcomed the new, it was hard to say goodbye to an old friend. I would have given most anything to have had Anna Belle by my side. Throughout that first year after her death, I buried my grief by doing her job and mine. I couldn't admit how much I sorely missed her and or how helpless I felt when she was ill.

And I will never hear Bette Midler's song, 'The Rose,' without thinking of Anna Belle.

She was truly a woman of class.

Chapter 9
Schemes and Scams
1990-1994

As wonderful as Linda and the other wealthy women had been to us, others were not so kind. Every non-profit has its share of horror stories; some are real nightmares and others are only mildly disappointing. When it comes to the world of fundraising events and the people who make them happen, personalities collide, egos dominate over mission, and some simply use the event for their own gain—or try to.

The Rose was no different. Most of those experiences are water so far under the bridge I can barely recall the people's faces. Yet, fair warning to new non-profits, there are times when the gift a donor brings isn't worth the price it will ultimately cost.

In the 1980s and early '90s, it was common for some donors to ask for documentation for their 'tax write-off,' stating that their gift was worth a whole bunch more than its value. It wasn't right, and the first time I said no, the donor's response created waves through an entire organization that had funded us.

I stood my ground. There simply wasn't any way I was going to document a donation of $10,000 for a pile of left over, mismatched tiles that were supposed to create the flooring throughout our second center. His workers had left the pile outside our doors. It stood nearly four feet high and covered two parking spaces. There wasn't enough of the same type of tiles in that mess to create a four by four entryway for the center. And to add insult to injury, we had to pay someone to have them carried off to the dump.

There was the time when I was attending a kick-off event for the annual luncheon held by an organization that had supported us in the past. The members were all so excited because they had a 'real' socialite who had agreed to chair it; someone who was well known in the community. I searched through the crowd for a familiar face, spied my friend Linda Strevell, and made my way over to stand next to her.

It was nearing 3 p.m., and we were gathered in the alcove of the Hotel Continental, with tables of finger food lined under and around the staircase. The crowd had spent the past hour tossing air kisses at each other, murmuring admirations at how good everyone looked, while balancing those tiny little plates filled with even tinier appetizers in one hand and holding a glass of wine in the other.

Finally the program began, and after a way too long introduction recounting the fame and success of the new chairperson, she stepped out onto the upper portion of a staircase in a rather grand style. When the applause stopped, she looked down on the crowd and gushed about the honor of being the chair, while reminding the group that she only agreed to chair the "best events" because her time was so valuable. Then she started describing the activities that were planned.

"We have secured the most prestigious country club in the city!" she announced. "It wasn't easy to retain the date I wanted. After all, you have to be a member, which fortunately I am, to even be able to have an event there." She smiled; a mouthful of pearly whites encouraged a round of nods from the crowd.

"Everyone who raises real money uses this country club, their service is superb and their food incredible. I was surprised you didn't have your luncheon there before." She looked pointedly at the past luncheon chairperson before continuing. "Our theme is Paris in the springtime, and we all know how beautiful that place is, especially in April—my husband insists on taking me there every year." She paused. "The luncheon will be the talk of the season!" More nods. "We have a fabulous raffle and our tickets will be $100 each." I heard a couple of gasps from the crowd, that amount was a little steep, even for this group.

"We already have commitments for the most fantastic items for the silent auction…" and she pulled out a sheet of paper and proceeded to read a list of exclusive places, theater events, certificates to expensive restaurants, and luxury items. Then she started describing the highlight of the silent auction—an exclusive dinner for ten, prepared in the lucky winner's home by Chef Ricardo, from a famous five-star local restaurant.

"I was so pleased that Ricardo agreed to do the dinner," she gushed, "he is the best chef in town and I don't know what we would have done without his support at my last event. What a coup it is to have him. I started to put his dinner as a raffle item but decided against that. We, the committee, were talking and realized that we couldn't possibly put it in the raffle." At this point she paused, and I swear she leaned in a bit, as if sharing some incredibly private confidence.

"I asked the committee, 'What would he do if the winning ticket was bought by someone from Deer Park?'" She laughed out loud, cocked her head, and said with a smirk, "I mean, what on earth could he cook for them? And imagine him going to Deer Park? Maybe he could make some barbecue…or something…"

The crowd came alive. Everyone laughed, everyone except me and Linda. I looked at her and she moved in closer to me and whispered, "I can't believe she just said that."

"I can't either," I answered between clenched teeth, feeling a wave of anger move up and over me.

"She can't know where Deer Park is or that it is so close to Pasadena or that Dr. Melillo is from Pasadena…" Linda's voice dropped another level. I couldn't stop staring at that woman standing on the landing in her too high heels and too expensive suit, and I wondered what it would take to knock that too smart smirk off her face.

Linda noticed the look on my face, gently took my arm and started moving me out of the middle of the crowd. By the time we reached the lobby, I was still fuming and she took my shoulders and turned me to face her.

"Dorothy," she said, her gaze boring into my eyes, "Wasn't Linda Hofheinz from Deer Park?" Her maneuver caught me off-guard and I had to smile.

"No, she was from Baytown but she taught school in Deer Park," I said.

Linda shrugged and said, "Lots of good folks come from Deer Park."

"And they don't all eat barbecue!" I added. We laughed, leaving as quickly as we could.

Another event was equally daunting.

Imagine my excitement at having a world famous author agree to host a fundraiser for The Rose in her 20,000 square foot home on the lake. It was beyond our every dream. I remember the night we all gathered at a restaurant to talk about the event. The two successful women, Jane the author and Dixie the general surgeon, sat next to each other. I was struck by the similarities between them, both were tall, both had these attractive chiseled faces with strong cheekbones and big blue eyes, each successful in her own right.

Dixie was going on about how she couldn't imagine living in such a big house as Jane's. "My little place is only 500 square feet, it sets back on fourteen acres but I couldn't afford a house that big."

There was something about the look on Jane's face and the tone in her voice when she said, "Of course you could, Dixie." She looked directly at Dixie, picked up a cigarette and lit it before finishing the thought. "If you didn't have twelve horses you could afford a big house just like mine. I know how expensive horses are to care for." Her voice was icy cold; her statement was not one of those 'joking on the square' comments. She flat out challenged Dixie's 'poor doctor' ruse and wasn't about to let it drop. She continued to question Dixie about horses and the cost of trainers and food, dropping in comments that every physician she knew made plenty of money. Dixie rose to her challenge, and suddenly they were engaged in a full-on fencing match.

I should have realized the competition between them would mean trouble for The Rose, but I didn't. Weeks passed as the planning continued. Kim, my right hand person, had printed and mailed invitations; news releases were sent and published.

I can't remember if the phone call came from one of the people we had invited or someone who had seen the news article, but I do remember the exact words she said: "There must be a mistake. The date of your event is the same night as the Art Center event at Jane's home. I don't think she'd be hosting both."

Frantic, with an awful sense of dread, I called our contact who was friends with the author. By the end of the day, we had the full story. Seems Ms. Author had recently become involved with the Art Center and been deeply moved by its work and inspired by its new male director. She decided she would rather have an event for them. She had changed her mind, plain and simple. There wasn't even an effort to suggest that she, or her assistant, had misunderstood the date, and no one offered to arrange another date for us. She simply decided that the mission of the arts was more in line with her work.

We were stunned. People told me we should have had a contract. Even today, if someone offered to open their home for a fundraiser, we wouldn't draw up a contract. Of course, we would have lots of emails to verify intents and offers, not just the verbal agreement.

There were other folks who used The Rose to their own advantage and forwarded their personal agenda. Sometimes they weren't fundraisers, but researchers who would try to convince me that having The Rose listed as a contributing organization, albeit on the final section of acknowledgements, was certainly worth the expense of our staff pulling hundreds of charts to look for the data they needed.

The Rose had built a data base of tremendous value; our population mirrored the ethnicity of Harris County, almost to the exact percentage: 38% Caucasian, 35% Hispanic, 19% Black, 5% Asian, and 2% other. Our group also reflected the overall younger age of our city. Yet its real value was that it included the full range of social economic measures coupled with geographic information. Having years of statistics for insured and uninsured women was a gold mine. The fact that we had also captured more than demographics and collected all kinds of health information made it even more valuable.

I got caught in that game once, allowing our resources to be used for someone's research paper as they pursued funding for their own programs. I swore we'd never do anything 'free' for the 'big guys' again. Yet, still they came, trying to reason with me.

One researcher exploded in my office when I flatly said no. Unless he would include $5 a chart in his National Cancer Institute budget, we weren't going to participate. His arguments fell on deaf ears and he stomped out slinging a parting insult, "They told me you were difficult to work with," he sneered, "and it's true."

You bet it is. Fool me once, shame on you…fool me twice…we all know the rest of that line.

Chapter 10
Stepping Up

The years between 1993 and 2000 were magical, miserable, and filled with more miracles than ever before. For The Rose, it was a time of major expansion. We moved into a real medical building, renting a 4,000 square foot office at the very end of the hall on the second story, which truth be known wouldn't pass fire codes with only one door in and out. That move marked a major transition in the life of The Rose.

At that time, one of the criticisms about The Rose was that it operated out of a 'storefront.' Since it wasn't located in a 'real' medical building, it therefore couldn't offer the 'best' service. (How odd that ten years later some of the major hospitals opened breast centers in storefronts.)

When we first moved into this real medical building from our tiny 988 square foot office, I thought, *We will never fill it up.* The amount of space was an incredible luxury. For the first time in six years I had an office all my own, so did a lot of other folks. There was a nice size waiting area, separate check-in and check-out counters, dedicated mammography and ultrasound rooms, a huge kitchen area that doubled as the staff meeting room, boardroom, and a place for the volunteers to gather and stuff envelopes or prepare patient charts. We still survived with donated furniture, a huge eight by eight wooden table filled most of the room, a gift from a cousin's work place. I loved that table, some of our best decisions were made sitting around it.

The sole purpose of moving to the larger space was to expand into diagnostic services and add ultrasound procedures and biopsies. Try as they might, our contacts at MD Anderson couldn't take our patients anymore; their policy had changed and they no longer accepted uninsured patients based on a "suspicious" mammogram. Their policy required that the patient only be accepted after obtaining a "documented diagnosis of cancer," which meant a pathology report.

We argued that if a woman could not scrape up $50 for a

mammogram, how the heck was she going to afford a diagnostic work-up? Ultrasound exams ranged from $150 to $300 at local hospitals, and an outpatient biopsy topped out at $1,000; add pathology and other clinical charges and the bill could easily run another $1,000. That was more money than most of our women made in two months. If we couldn't get the diagnosis, we sure couldn't get surgery or treatment for those women.

Even though Dixie had always been able to convince Bayshore Medical Center to let her do a few surgeries at no charge, there were limits. We were running out of options for our sponsored patients, and helplessly watched as one patient after another was turned away by the charity hospitals. The public health system was no help, even if the women lived in Harris County. It took over eleven months for women to get through the system, and for some of our women that wait was a death sentence.

We also needed to expand services if we hoped to keep our paying patients. Gone were the days of only doing $50 mammograms and handling payments on a cash basis. We had entered the world of accepting insurance and becoming a provider for managed care plans. Getting approved by both insurance and managed care was a lengthy process requiring tons of paperwork. Being a specialty service was a handicap in itself and eliminated any bargaining power. But we had no choice, we were losing too many patients because we didn't take insurance.

Finding the new location had taken months, completing the build out even longer, it had been a tough transition. It was also a huge step financially. Our rent alone was half of the previous year's entire budget, but we had worked out a deal and obtained several months free rent. Enough time, we reasoned, for us to get our biopsy program going strong. We needed equipment, space, supplies, a physician on-site capable of doing them, and a pathologist to report on them. Dixie could do some of our procedures, but she still had a full-time practice to run, so our radiologist, Dr. K., had to learn.

"Dorty, I need a cow boop." Dr. K. stood in front of my desk, impatiently shifting her weight from one foot to the other. I glanced up at her. The look on her face was dead serious. She was an excellent radiologist but she had a talent of creating the best of times and the worst of times at The Rose. I studied her, silently debating which one she would be creating today.

Her oversized lab coat dwarfed her tiny frame and gaped open haphazardly. When she sped down the hall the tails of it would swing from side to side, out of sync with her jackrabbit pace. But eccentricities aside, few radiologists could equal Dr. K. in detecting early cancers; she had one of the best eyes in the business.

She stood in front of me waiting, hands on her hips, her dark eyes snapping at me. Random sections of her short coal black hair refused to be tamed by hairspray and stood out at odd points around her face. There were times when she had the look of a mad scientist, and this was definitely one of them.

"A what, Dr. K? You need a what?" I asked.

"A cow boop. You know what I mean," she bent over halfway, pushed her elbows out, and with her hands made a circular motion around the area of her chest. "A cow boop, where the milk comes from, I need it to practice on." Her Asian-accented speech clipped words, sometimes making a conversation an experiment in itself.

"You mean an udder. You want me to find you a cow's udder? A dead cow's udder?" I was accustomed to being on the receiving end of unreasonable requests from radiologists, but this was one of the better ones.

"Yes, so I can do the biopsy, I need to practice on it."

"Aren't you supposed to use turkey breasts for that?" I questioned, praying this conversation would end soon. She usually didn't give up, an image of a bull dog's mouth chomping down on my butt floated up in front of me.

"It's not the same." She had her arguments ready, "The bweast of our patients are tough. It takes a lot to push the tip of the needle in the skin to the leeson." She made this weird motion with her hands, one hand cupped against and under the other as she mimicked the turning of a screwdriver. "And our patients' boops are big, no one is like those turkeys, they have big boops like the cows."

"Can't we just go out and buy you bigger turkey breasts?" I pleaded. I knew attempting reason with this woman was futile, but ever the optimist, I plugged on.

"No! Bigger turkey won't work. It is the texture, the tissue is stringy." She rubbed her thumb against the tips of her fingers. "That is why I want the boop, its texture is like woman's." She folded her arms across her chest. She really was serious.

"Dr. K., where would I find a cow boop?" a final whine, a desperate plea for mercy slipped from my lips.

"You will find it. If you want me to do the biopsies, I need the cow boop." With that she turned on one heel and was out the door.

I dropped my head to my hands and just stared at the desk. Sixty thousand dollars of equipment, a new ultrasound machine, a bioptic gun and all the surgical supplies for the ultrasound biopsy program were being delivered that week. Everything we had planned was in place.

Now it all hinged on a cow boob.

"A cow boob," I corrected myself. "Where on earth will I find that?" I said to the walls, halfway expecting an answer.

From someone who has cows. The thought drifted in from nowhere.

Reminding myself that hearing voices was a reactionary phenomenon, usually temporary, resulting from times of unrelenting stress and not a definite symptom of insanity, I picked up the phone and called my cousin Brad.

Everyone should have a cousin Brad. In fact, everyone should be lucky enough to be part of a family like the Perrys. Every now and then, when I'm at one of the annual family reunions, I find myself musing and trying to establish the blood line between us. Then I remember we are cousins by marriage, cousins once or twice removed at that. Sure, I'm biased, but there's not been a step along the way of The Rose's journey that some member of that family wasn't right there beside me, willing to help, be it cousin Helen or her boys Brad and Chris or any of the others. This time was no different.

Brad didn't even laugh when I asked if he could get me a cow udder. His response was low and even. You'd have thought I'd asked him to pick up bread and milk on his way home from work.

"Not sure when I'll get back over to the slaughter house. You know that's where I'll have to go to find one. How soon do you need it?" he asked. Before I could answer, he lumbered on, "If I'd known you needed one, I would have picked it up when I was there two weeks ago. Did you hear that Dad and I got a five pointer? Yep, be a lot of good meat from that one. They might not have one you know, the cow udder; I may have to ask them to save me one. It's about forty minutes away, north on 59, that's the only slaughter house in the area. I know them well, that's where we took all Crystal's pigs. Did Mom tell you about coming up for the pig sale? We all met last weekend in Brenham and stayed at a bed and breakfast. It was a really nice place." I was ready to interrupt and try to get him back on track when he said, "Guess I could come and get you when I get off work on Thursday." Brad worked nights for the railroad. He lived in Cleveland, about seventy miles north of town. He and Sandra, with daughters Crystal and Brettney, raised cows, pigs, and a few horses. "You do want to go with me?" he added innocently.

"No!" I exclaimed, squirming in my chair, breaking out into a sweat, hoping that wasn't going to be part of the deal. "Please don't make me do that! Remember, I'm a city girl."

Only then did I hear the chuckle in his voice. "The things I do for you," he laughed out loud, and hung up after promising to get me one before the week was out.

Brad keeps his promises. A few days later, he walked into my office carrying a medium-sized ice chest.

"Where do you want it?" he asked, and I guided him and it down the hall, keeping my distance, hoping no one would follow us into the kitchen. He set it on the table and opened the top. I looked down. Sure enough, there was a cow's udder nestled in ice.

"What do I owe you?"

"Nothing," he grinned, "you can buy me lunch one day and we'll call it even. I know how much you hate going out to lunch but that's the price," he laughed and then added, "What is it you're needing this for again?"

I started to explain but stopped and reached for the phone. In my most professional tone, my voice went out over the intercom. "Dr. K., please report to the staff area for training."

I would let her explain it to him. That conversation took up the rest of the morning.

It was about that time when I hired a person who would change the course of The Rose forever. Louise was a redhead, freckles, green eyes, the whole package. Her small frame carried an ample body; she wasn't heavy by any means, but standing a shade under five feet tall would never allow her to be described as svelte.

She reminded me of an elf, all playful and perky with a sense of urgency entering into every conversation. Her hands stayed in constant motion when she spoke and her smile, broad and wide, could melt any heart. She had a way of never finishing a sentence, moving from one idea to the other and filling the gaps in between with bits and pieces of a quirky unique humor.

She was a natural counselor and a good writer, and sought us out for a part-time grant writing job. Diagnosed nine years previously, she knew how it felt hearing the words "You have breast cancer," and she knew the emotional and physical demands involved in surgery and chemotherapy. She had wrestled with the disbelief of her own mortality and had fought against the fear created by every new ache or potential symptom.

At this stage in her life, she really didn't need to work, her husband made more than enough for their support. She had grown kids and grandkids, had just completed a counselor's degree and was thinking about entering a Master's program in ministerial work. But, she confided, she needed work to feel useful and worthwhile.

Twenty hours a week at $10 an hour was all she wanted and more than we could afford, but I needed the help badly. Back in those days, all of the grant writing and grant reporting fell to me. That year I would raise over a million dollars through grants. No small sum when considering it represented nearly one half of our total budget.

Louise was the first real grant writer we ever hired. Although logically I knew it was a good move to bring her on board, I struggled with the time it took to bring her up to speed and on most days found it more trouble than it was worth. Just the process of explaining how things worked at The Rose, infusing her with the information needed for her to write those compelling stories, trying to help her understand the impact of the revenue from paying women, all of it was extra work for me. I had enough to do with handling the day-to-day operations, trying to manage employees and physicians, and looking for funds to cover the constant need for more equipment and more staff.

She didn't need any tutoring to understand the breast cancer journey, but she knew it from an insured woman's point of view. It took weeks for her to fully accept the lack of choices for the uninsured.

Louise believed, as did most folks, that anyone diagnosed with breast cancer, insured or not, could go to MD Anderson and their care would be exactly the same as she had received. She couldn't comprehend that most uninsured women did not go to MD Anderson or to any other major cancer center. Most had to go through the public health systems, UTMB in Galveston if the woman lived outside of Harris County, or Harris County Hospital system for those in-county residents. They really did not have a choice in treatment, the majority—over 90% at that time—had a mastectomy and chemotherapy. It was the most cost effective way to go—from the facility's perspective and the woman's. Few of our sponsored women could afford to take the time off work that was needed for radiation therapy, two hours every day, five days a week for six weeks, and without radiation therapy, conservative surgery was out of the question.

I learned later that her perceived inability to grasp the situation of the uninsured was because she was one of those soft-hearted folks who empathized so deeply that she had trouble disengaging herself from the women she was writing about. Her constant questioning and disbelief fought her growing understanding that the grim reality of being poor and uninsured almost guaranteed late stage diagnosis, which translated into early death.

"But I don't understand, Dorothy." She sat across from me, fussing with the scarf that draped over her shoulders. "Anyone can go to MD Anderson. It's a state-supported charity, that's why it is there, to take care of the uninsured."

"No they can't, Louise. The hospital's guidelines for charity care are for the really poor—which means a person cannot make more than $3,000 a year. Those are the only ones who get in if they live in Harris

County. Most of our uninsured women are working, so they make $8,000-10,000 a year."

"How can anyone live on $10,000 a year?" she asked, the sharpness in her voice conveyed a sense of outrage. She knew it was a question that had no answers. Then she would turn on the other local charity hospitals. "But everyone *thinks* they care for the poor, isn't that why they can raise so many millions of dollars?"

Here we go again, I thought, and I would try to explain how the system really worked.

Women living in Harris County went to Ben Taub or LBJ, where physicians from Baylor or MD Anderson would oversee their care. For the rest of the state, it was UTMB in Galveston. Those are the only systems. A few non-profit hospitals, like St. Joseph, offered care, but the request had to be made by an internal doctor.

She argued that it wasn't "right." The "it" ranged from the fact that uninsured women didn't have the option of breast conservation or reconstruction to major cancer centers not having to provide care and the myths that abounded around the availability of charity care and cancer treatment.

She pushed on, "I saw a presentation the other night at church about the number of indigent that MD Anderson takes care of—it was an amazing number. How can they say that?"

"Their Medicaid patients are counted in the indigent care. Add to that the care their physicians provide to thousands at the public hospital," I said. "Look, I'm not criticizing them. They do provide an amazing amount of care, and remember, we are able to get the wild types of cancers into them without a lot of hassle, those cancers that are especially aggressive or in younger women."

That really set her off and I braced myself for spending yet another half-hour of discussion and explanation.

It was Louise and her questioning that marked a major turning point in the life of The Rose.

"Didn't you help Dixie found The Rose?"

"Yes, of course I did," I replied, annoyed at another question. Louise knew our history.

"Then why aren't you mentioned anywhere in the grant proposals or any of the press releases?"

I wasn't in a very good mood that day and I had grown a little sensitive to her criticism. We had different writing styles, and she was convinced hers was superior to mine, which sometimes it was. I jumped to the conclusion that this line of questioning was just another ploy to change some text in a grant proposal.

"Why would I be?" I asked, "Especially when Dixie's story is so compelling. Think about it—here we have a high school dropout who becomes doctor, and is in fact the second female to complete surgical residency at UTMB. She was kicked out of high school because she was pregnant, and against all odds went back to college then medical school. What a story! She went on to become a champion for breast cancer care. I've always been amazed at how open she is with her patients! She was one of the first doctors to share her phone number with patients. She's a symbol of everything that is needed in medicine. And she went beyond the doctoring part, she started The Rose…"

"But only because you helped her," Louise interrupted. "You were there from the very beginning." She added, "Dixie told me that if it weren't for you there wouldn't be a Rose." A question mark slowly covered her face; she waited patiently for me to reply. I looked back at her, still wondering where in the world this conversation was headed.

"Dorothy, you are the co-founder of The Rose, not just the executive director of it!" Her words were a proclamation. "You are as responsible as Dixie for its existence. You ran it while working full time at Bayshore, you wrote the grants that gave it the funds for equipment. You even put in your own money to get it going."

I laughed. "That's true, but my 'investment' was small compared to Dixie's, for the attorney's fee to file the IRS application."

"A form that YOU completed—not him!" She almost hissed the words as she leaned forward. "And tell me, what did that $400 mean to you? Wasn't that when your husband wasn't working? How much were you earning compared to Dixie?"

I didn't answer, shaking my head. That $400 was my total savings, but that wasn't anyone's business.

"Didn't you leave your job and all the benefits to run this place? You committed just as much to The Rose as anyone, and it's time to share that fact. You need to be listed alongside Dixie as co-founder on The Rose letterhead and in every story."

"I really don't see the point, Louise."

"You don't now, but you will. Who is it that is doing all the presentations these days? Who is it that responds to every media call? Who is it that is interviewed on TV or radio? Not Dixie. You and I both know she's too busy and…" and she paused, those hands moved nervously in front of her, she looked away for a moment, before continuing, "…the truth is she doesn't really want to do the talks anymore and hates being on TV."

I felt the heat rise in my face and answered with, "You know how many calls we are receiving, most of them asking for her. She has to keep her practice going. She has to draw a line somewhere. It's my job to fill in for her. Everyone wants her to be the speaker…" I struggled, sounding more and more defensive.

"That's not totally true anymore," Louise stopped me, her words direct. "Honestly, Dorothy, while folks may know of her, what they want to hear about is The Rose."

I felt as uncomfortable as she looked. Dixie had always been the prominent figure, the only person we promoted with the story of The Rose. After all, she was the visionary, the founder. Well, the co-founder. I was a worker bee, the behind-the-scenes person, the one who led from the shadows. It had always been important to me to keep Dixie in the forefront. It was a system that had worked well, until now.

"Face it, Dorothy. The Rose isn't just Dixie's organization, it's yours too!" she chewed at her lip, then added softly, "It may be more yours than hers. She will always be a doctor first, and that's okay," she smiled. "But if The Rose is going to move forward, it's going to be up to you!" Her words hung in the air.

"In this proposal, I changed your title to co-founder and added your part to the history of The Rose." She handed me the draft. "You are the leader of The Rose. You can't stay in the background any longer. It's time for you to accept your place in this story."

"But…" I started.

She frowned, pursed her lips, and shook her head so hard that her short red hair bounced from side to side. I had seen that look before and knew Louise's mind was made up.

"Just read it and trust me on this one." She stood up, reached out and tapped the stack of papers, "And, don't go changing the part about you, leave it alone." She left the room with a swish.

I looked down at the sheets of paper and slowly started to read her words. They forced me back to our beginning and I was lost in that time, remembering all the days and nights of uncertainty, all the challenges, all the hopes and the dreams.

We seldom shared those early hardships, at least not publicly. Like the time the only way for The Rose to replace a mammogram machine was with a personal guarantee of its financing. Dixie knew better than to agree to that kind of arrangement, but I signed anyway. I was too naïve not to, and we had to have that machine.

For the past ten years, it was always a struggle, from finding enough funding to keep up with ever-advancing imaging systems, to working with antiquated patient tracking and data systems, to having enough paid patients to offset the costs of the unpaid.

I was embarrassed that it had taken so long to offer medical benefits to employees, and thought about how I had daily prayed that no one would get sick or get divorced and lose their husband's coverage. What we paid in salaries was at the bottom of the line, far from even being remotely competitive. All we had to offer our employees as we tried to hang on to the good ones or recruit new ones was the reward of doing this good work and the dream of 'someday.'

Tears filled my eyes. But instead of blurring my vision they made the words and sentences come into focus even sharper and clearer.

Soon all the letterhead was changed to reflect the names of the "Co-Founders." The narrative for our history was permanently amended on every brochure, in all proposals, in each telling and retelling of the story of The Rose. Such seemingly minor changes would carry a huge impact in the years to come.

Chapter 11
The Courage to Change

In spite of Louise's insistence, accepting my public role within The Rose did not come easily, but the change started during a trip to Bermuda. It was March, 1997, and Dixie had convinced me to go with her to another of those four-day medical meetings.

She needed the CMEs and the location was luxurious. There was an additional enticement—it was paid for in its entirety by one of the pharmaceutical companies. They agreed to cover my fare as well as Dixie's attendance.

Bermuda is a beautiful island with a magical green mountainous countryside dipping down into the deepest blue ocean. Landscapes are covered with colorful foliage, pink tiled roofs sparkle in the endless sunshine, and everywhere are the reminders of a former, more elegant British heritage.

Try as I might, I couldn't be excited about this trip. I was grateful…truly. Traveling to such a gorgeous place was a rare treat for me.

But once again, I was in a place I didn't want or need to be. I was up to my shoulders in problems at work, coping with a home life that had turned miserable, and worried about bills at both places. Running a struggling non-profit that consumed fifteen hours of every day and always needed more—more funding, more equipment, more patients—was the overarching focus of life. After twelve years of these annual pilgrimages, I had heard all the major players lecture multiple times and, from a lay person's point of view, found the presentations redundant and tedious. The days of these journeys being exciting were long gone.

If I were totally honest I would have to admit that going on a trip outside the United States terrified me. This trip to Bermuda was the first time I had boarded a plane in a year. That last trip had ended in a nightmare that left me crippled for months.

Usually the conferences were in the mainland United States, but last year the venue was Hawaii. "It is the trip of a lifetime!" Dixie had exclaimed. She had it all planned out, she'd take her son Ralph and I would take Alan and we'd turn it into a real vacation. It didn't take much to convince me to go. The room rates were cheap, and flights were so incredibly low even I could afford them.

The seminar was uneventful but the afternoons of sightseeing were amazing. On the very last day, Alan and I left our room at dawn, hoping to catch the morning journey of the whales. We walked across the dewy, lush green lawns, empty of people, and breathed in the flower scented cool morning air. I thanked God for another day in paradise.

I looked out over the huge expanse of water ahead of us, shimmering with golden hues from the rising sun, and congratulated myself for keeping our expenses in check. At the very moment that thought left my mind, I felt my right leg sinking. I was falling. Somewhere in the near distance I heard a snapping sound, and in the next moment I was flat out on the ground.

Stunned, I tried to get up and pulled myself to a sitting position. I stared down at my leg, thinking I had twisted my ankle, but my right foot hung cockeyed at an angle to the leg. There was no way I could move it. At that point, I didn't feel any pain, only a sense that something incredibly bad had just happened. Something I was helpless to fix.

Alan stared at my foot, yelped out loud at the sight, and said, "Stay here, I'll get help." He ran back up to the resort, and I thought, *Where could I go?* Fear gripped my insides and I tried to focus but I couldn't quit staring at my foot, dangling and limp, held only by stretched tendons and skin.

Then it started to throb and pain seared through my being.

I'd like to say that the next 72 hours were a blur, that the medication when it was finally administered in the ambulance moved me to la-la land, but that isn't true. By the time the EMT folks arrived, the pain was in full force, gripping my being with such intensity that the memory of it still sets my teeth on edge. I was too shocked to scream, my mouth wouldn't function and I fought to stay alert as waves of agony moved over me.

I remember being lifted onto the stretcher, the incredibly long journey through the manicured lawns to reach the front of the building and driveway. I remember the screaming sirens, morphine being pushed into my arms, now the waves of pain were mixed with waves of nausea. I felt every bump in the road as the vehicle sped to the hospital. I remember being in the emergency room, being wheeled to x-ray, more morphine going in my arm, and breaking down in sobs when I saw Dixie. She was talking with the ER doctor.

All three of my ankle bones were broken. Lucky for me, it was a clean snap. The hole I had stepped in was where a water meter resided, sunk deep into the ground. I remember people saying the resort should have had it gated or fenced off. I remember talk of the resort's liability, discussions of surgery, of pins and plates and me asking the question: Would I walk again?

Having the surgery in Hawaii was not an option. I sure couldn't afford the premium rates for Alan to stay and I didn't want to be alone. I wasn't even sure what the insurance would cover, we had taken the cheapest group policy we could manage for employees. I wanted Dr. Heisey back in the States to do my surgery. He was the best. What I wanted more than anything was to go home.

Dixie finally convinced the attending physician that, as a general surgeon, she could manage me. She could certainly give me pain medicine, and she vouched that I had the will power to make the seventeen-hour plane ride home in an open cast. It turned out to be a lot more than seventeen hours but I managed. Later Dixie told me she had no idea if I'd make it or not, but she sure wasn't leaving me there. Thank God. I don't know what I would have done without Dixie.

They secured my leg in an air cast and transferred me via ambulance to the airport. Dixie and Ralph maneuvered my wheelchair through the airport corridors, skirting security and dodging idiot people who nearly ran into my leg, which stuck straight out, bandaged and swollen. We started the long journey home. Alan walked beside me in a daze, looking as helpless as I felt.

The airline agreed to move me to a vacant seat in the front row of first class to accommodate my cast, but that change had to be paid at the current first class rate, adding another $1,000 to the bill. No matter how Alan and Dixie reasoned with them, there was no budging. They had sold the seat I had originally paid for, and even then didn't discount my 'new' fare. In the end, I'm sure they wished they had insisted on an even higher fare, especially after I spent most of those hours in the air throwing up. The sounds, smells, and sight of my condition were obviously making all the first class passengers feel queasy. Some ignored my retching, pulling their magazines or papers close to their face, others openly stared at me with disdain; one asked the stewardess if I could be moved.

The next year was filled with surgeries, learning to walk on crutches, hard cast, soft cast, ankle air cast, canes, ice boots and rehab. It took two days after landing before the swelling was brought under control and the first surgery could be done. Pins and plates secured the bones back together. Six months later there was another surgery to take the pins and plates out, the bones had healed well but during the process the hardware had shifted, creating another type of unrelenting pain.

After the first two weeks of recovery, I started working from home, editing and finishing the first *Rose Cookbook*. It was another fundraising project that we were sure would bring in tons of money. Of course, it was only modestly successful, but at the time we had high hopes for it. Every day, volunteers came and went as we worked on the layout and copy. Employees brought me paperwork that needed my signature and I wrote grant proposals on my home computer.

My house was built with a 'mother-in-law' apartment, which is where I set up shop; my days spent trying to concentrate between times of lucidity and doses of pain medicine. Everyone, my employees, my volunteers, my friends, neighbors engulfed me in concern and caring, everyone except my husband.

Maybe he took it as a sign that I could manage without help when I started working on the cookbook. Maybe he honestly thought I was okay. Maybe he didn't think at all. But three weeks after being released from the hospital, with me still wheelchair bound, he announced he would be gone for the entire day, he had to play golf. He had committed to this tournament a long time ago and he was the best player on the team, they couldn't get along without him.

I was crushed but much too proud to object. For a guy who didn't have a job, it never ceased to amaze me that he could justify the cost of playing golf. But I didn't argue, I didn't have the strength.

Somewhere around midday, I heard a noise coming from the other room. Someone was knocking at the side door and then tried to open it. My heart was beating hard, I was immediately on guard.

No one was scheduled to visit that day and solicitors usually came to the front door. My ever-faithful companion, Saucy dog, growled, deep and menacingly, her ears standing straight up. Nearing 100 pounds, Saucy could be frightening, but even with her protection, I feared we were about to be robbed. Daytime burglaries had recently plagued our neighborhood, which was set off the main road and filled with old-timers or homebound residents. The pickings were ripe. I knew a determined robber would think nothing of killing a dog, or me.

The rattling of the door knob continued, followed by a hard push on the door. The extra lock held. Saucy leapt into action, her bark fierce and loud, running into the other room. Moments passed. She continued to bark then stopped. All was silent. Whoever was at the door was gone.

Returning to me, with her giant tail wagging, she nuzzled her wet nose against my hand, trying to unclench it from the wheel of the chair. She whimpered. It's okay now, she signaled, looking up at me. The danger is over.

Yes, it's over. I took a deep breath, still trembling from the fear, begging my heart to slow down and convincing my bladder it didn't really have to go to the bathroom. I couldn't even manage that task alone very easily.

Over, I thought, *the same is true for this marriage.* It had been on the rocks for a long time. *Just let me get back on my feet again and I won't put up with this any longer,* I promised myself.

This was the first time as an adult that I had not been able to walk or care for myself. A month later, I would celebrate my forty-eighth birthday by walking with crutches and fully returning to work.

After our radiologist assured me I would never wear heels or dance again, I assured her with equal confidence that she was wrong. My daily visualizations included me dancing in red high heels. I couldn't walk yet, but I would dance. No matter how hard the day, or how much the pain, I never let Alan see me cry. Someone who cared more about a day of golf would never see me sad again.

So there I was in Bermuda, almost a year to the day after the accident in Hawaii, far from home and feeling sad. In fact, I was close to anger. Somehow this trip needed to be fun for me too.

Dixie never liked to leave the hotel after the meetings, but I loved exploring the city and seeing new things. Throughout the years, I had volunteered to go for beer, wine, and Tab runs, and while out I would work in my own version of sightseeing. In Miami, I got caught up in a street riot. In Los Angeles, I walked for blocks, enjoying the endless flowers of April. Bermuda was no exception. I wanted to see something of the island, go on an adventure and test the strength of my ankle. So I climbed to the top of the hill from our resort, found an old historic lighthouse and enjoyed the tour guide's stories.

It wasn't until late afternoon, on my way back down the hill, that I realized I was in trouble; my ankle was swelling, badly. I didn't carry a cell phone, and I became a little more lost with every step.

As I hobbled down the hill, more annoyed at myself than anything else, I wondered what the heck I was doing there. My little excursion had been the only highlight of the week and it was quickly turning into a disaster. Off in the distance, I spotted a taxi. Moving as fast as I dared, I waved my arms over my head, yelled loudly and breathed a sigh of relief when the car turned toward me.

As luck would have it, I wasn't far from the resort but the route I was on would have taken me two streets north of it, meaning I would have totally missed it. My ankle was swollen, my foot hurt, my leg ached. The seminar was over for the day and I caught up with Dixie. That evening other doctors joined us; there was lots of conversation and dinner. I barely mentioned the near misadventure.

The next morning I sat through meeting after meeting, despairing that it was only 9:30 a.m. With four long hours yet to go, I started to journal in my trusty spiral notebook. I knew there would be no escape for me on that day, no walks, no sightseeing, not with my ankle still swollen double.

That's when it happened.

I watched as the words flooded the pages, angry words, thoughts I had never dared admit to before. My emotions were so sharp they gouged deep holes in my most tender places. I couldn't stop writing, bold black ink filled up line after line. Sentences describing feelings, observations, and self-questioning covered page after page. While the speakers droned on, my pen never stopped. At one point Dixie asked me what I was writing and I responded it was just stuff for work.

But it wasn't. I was deeply involved in producing my new manifesto, and it was one that meant all things had to change.

Listening to the doctors talk the previous night had triggered something in me, something I had never felt before. Dixie's stories were always outrageously funny and normally had me in stitches. One of her favorites was about women coming to her wanting hormones. "I tell them if I was married to some old codger who had a big old gut and an old smelly cigar hanging out of his mouth, I wouldn't want to have sex with him either. It's not about sex drive, it's about the person!" She confided to the others, "I tell my patients what they need is some good looking young guy, and when they get someone like that, they sure won't need any hormones!"

Everyone laughed and the debate about hormones started up. Dixie had been against hormones for a long time and national studies were confirming her wisdom.

The more they talked, the more I realized that what they were saying wasn't so funny. My mouth fell open when I heard the comment about hormones being prescribed only for those women who were "too fat and lazy to exercise or eat right."

I was one of those women who took hormones. Menopause had been hard on me. Hot flashes were awful, came often, and were a very real issue. I was the same as all the other business women I knew who were dealing with menopause, muddling through board meetings and presentations trying to ignore the obvious flush and sweat popping out on my face. That agony alone was enough, but all the other symptoms made life miserable: nights without sleep, sweating so much the sheets were soaked, and the mood swings! Lord, who could ever be prepared for someone going from Little Bo Peep to Godzilla in a single stroke? Add bursting into tears, the unreasonable rage and bouts of depression, and, finally, I gave in and tried hormones. It wasn't a lot of help but it was something.

But on that night, listening to the docs talk, I didn't have the courage to object to the "fat and lazy" statement, I just seethed. Then outrage started to build in my soul. I always knew I was an outsider, yet I couldn't believe the course the conversation had taken.

The idea that women simply had to endure hot flashes was one thing, but thinking about all the breast cancer survivors who couldn't even find relief with hormones was another.

Chemotherapy throws most women into menopause, with every symptom that goes with it. But the evidence is clear, and the strong link between estrogen and breast cancer meant hormones were not an answer.

The fact that there was not one single effective alternative to hormones was, and still is, outrageous. It was another failure of modern medicine and more evidence that women's health was relegated to second place. To me, it was no less serious than the fact that more women died of their first heart attack than did men—mainly because 95% of all the research had been done on men.

So I seethed and listened, too timid and too much of a coward to object to their opinions.

Then the topic got around to marriage and relationships. Dixie said she had no need for a man to mess up her life or dirty up her house, and if she did find one, he sure couldn't be her age or older. "Why would I want to have to take care of some doddering old idiot for the rest of my life?" she'd ask. Heads nodded in agreement.

There was a time I held similar beliefs about men; I had been a big time male-basher. But on that night I realized I didn't feel that way anymore. The years had worn me down. Even though I wasn't in a good marriage, in my heart of hearts I still believed in romance. Watching so many women lose their battles to breast cancer while their husbands stood by, more afraid of losing them than the women were afraid of dying, had made a mark on my soul.

Sure, there was always the scoundrel who "didn't bargain for cancer" and who would abandon the woman, sometimes leaving her with kids to care for. But those were the exceptions, most of the husbands in our support groups were in unimaginable pain and heartbreak.

I knew love existed. I had seen it. And for whatever reason, my entire belief system about relationships, marriage and men, in fact, about life itself and most of all about The Rose, was being retooled and rerouted.

On that night in a bar hundreds of miles away from home, I realized I had to change. And if I couldn't find that courage soon, I would lose this dream of The Rose, and worse than that, I would lose 'me.'

Dixie had her practice and her patients. Louise was right, Dixie didn't want to do the presentations anymore and she didn't want to ask folks for donations. The Rose was a place where she could care for her patients, and that was what she wanted. No criticism, just fact.

She had set clear boundaries in her life; when she left for the day, her horses and her ranch had her full attention. She had a practice, she had The Rose when she needed it, and most of all she had a life outside both. Her priorities were clear.

What The Rose needed was a leader, not someone doing it part time or someone who was content to stay in the shadows of another person.

It was time I took the reins fully and got on with it. I could handle the public speaking; heck, I had done enough of it when I was on the management training faculty for Hospital Corporation of America, and I had been a darn good presenter. Even though I could recite Dixie's talk by rote, I soon learned that the talk about breast cancer and its symptoms wasn't the only thing people wanted to hear.

People loved the story of The Rose; they loved hearing how we started and why we continued. The Rose was becoming a big part of the wellbeing of our community.

So on that fateful morning, as I sat in a huge auditorium with my leg propped up and the voice of another boring speaker droning on in the background, I wrote down one goal after another. The sentences were punctuated with exclamation marks and words were underlined.

"No more going to physician seminars" was first on the list. Any workshops I attended in the future would be about non-profit management and fundraising. My next goals were building a new board of directors capable of raising funds and finding a full-time person to replace Louise (who had moved away). I had to stop being the only grant writer. I would recruit another radiologist. I would secure more funders.

Somewhere on the list was a sentence about resolving the marriage issues and allowing myself to let go of that burden. I remember blinking back the tears as I reread that sentence and wished for...for what? I couldn't find the words so I returned to the list for work. It was a long list.

In the year ahead, a lot of those goals became reality and our work transformed. The Rose grew stronger. The number of uninsured women needing screening and diagnosis exploded. The funding was always tricky but new donors came to help.

Each time I read a thank you note from a patient, listened to grateful family members or watched my staff move mountains when we had a difficult case—doing whatever it took to get a woman diagnosed and into treatment—all those events, big and small, moved me forward.

Finding my own voice didn't happen overnight, but not having one was no longer an option. I had a job to get done.

Chapter 12
A Matter of Money

By mid-1997, after Dr. K had moved on, our daily mantra was that we needed a full-time, on-site radiologist. Without one, our diagnostic program would come to a halt.

We thought we had found her replacement and ended up being badly burned by a guy who worked with us part time and convinced us he wanted to be part of The Rose full time. I'll never forget him picking up his contract and telling us he'd return it by Monday. He left saying his greatest dream was to be a "real partner" in our mission.

All the time he was talking to us, he was negotiating the deal he really wanted with a major medical system, using our offer, now in writing, as leverage. It would be one of many times when we reminded ourselves of the truth in the saying 'You knew it was a snake when you picked it up.'

After months of working with locum tenums, high dollar doctors hired from staffing agencies to work a day or a week or more, we found a female radiologist who looked like she would be a perfect match.

It was a Monday morning, one of those days in the life of The Rose that would turn our world inside out.

I was unloading my briefcase when Verlyn walked into my office. True to the promise to myself in Bermuda, I had hired a full-time grant writer and development person, but on days like this day I questioned my judgment.

"I have just seen the most gorgeous man," she said as she perched her left hip on the side of my desk, "he had the most gorgeous blue eyes." She paused and stared out of the window with a kind of dreamy look on her face.

"Verlyn, what are you talking about?" I asked.

"Just now," she answered slowly, "as I was getting off the elevator he was getting on." Verlyn had a distinctive voice. She spoke in a refined manner, obviously enjoyed stretching her vocabulary prowess, and she had a knack of controlling most conversations by moderating the pace of her words.

"Who was getting on?" I didn't wait for her reply. We had a full day ahead and a grant deadline to meet. "Have you finished the Texas Cancer Council proposal yet?"

"Didn't you see him? You must have." She ignored my question about the grant. Thick jet black hair framed a very attractive face; her dress was borderline sexy, nothing overt, simply the clinging of soft material in just the right places. No, it was her mannerisms, the toss of her head that made her hair swing or the hand seductively placed on her hip that emphasized her femininity. She was extremely creative, did a good job as my development director, but drove me crazy by going off on different tangents. Today she was talking about the UPS man while my only concern was getting the grant finished and out the door.

"Verlyn, could we get to work on the proposal? It's pretty darn important. Remember? Proposal? Your job?" My words were measured.

With a half laugh, she tossed out, "You know, Dorothy, you're just no fun at all."

I dismissed her with a shake of the head. She threw me a condescending grin, rolled her eyes and left. *She's right,* I thought, *I am no fun.* Before I had time to consider why, Olga stood at my door.

"Dorothy, do you have a minute? Do you remember Ms. Gonzales?" she asked.

"Who?"

"She was the lady that we diagnosed last June, the one who we had to keep working on…it took over two months…to get her to come back in for her biopsy. Remember, her son was getting married and she had to take care of everything for his wedding. So we kept rescheduling her biopsy. The pathology was positive."

"Last June? What's happened?"

She handed me Ms. Gonzales's chart and I reviewed the pages, sponsorship application, procedures reports, pathology report: positive, bilateral breast cancer.

"Where did she get treatment?" I asked, trying to put together this patient's story. I looked up at Olga. She was small framed, wore her dark hair short, her skin was fair.

She shifted her weight, looked away, and then said, "That's just it, Dorothy, she didn't."

Her precise words were laced with an accent different from the local Tex Mex dialect. Olga was from Columbia. Her speech had a rhythmic cadence and her words were heavy, rich with passion. I had to listen carefully.

"What? Tell me that again. No treatment? But it is February."

Olga continued, "You can see in the chart all the times I tried to reach her."

I scanned the form listing patient notes. There were a dozen plus entries, showing no answers, left messages, phone temporarily disconnected. Olga reached over my hands and pulled out other pieces of paper, saying, "Here are copies of the letters, both in English and Spanish, and the stubs showing we sent them registered. Today, for some reason I took a chance and called that same number. Ms. Gonzales answered."

"And?"

"She never had treatment. She said she had gone to the clinic like we told her. She understood she had to fill out the forms to be approved for Ben Taub and get her eligibility card. In fact, she went to the clinic five times, and each time they sent her away, wanting some different kind of paperwork or proof of residency or something. She doesn't drive, so a friend was taking her."

"She never got treatment?" I repeated. "Did she show them the pathology report?"

"Yes, she said she did. She said she told them she had a biopsy but they wouldn't approve her."

"I don't believe this." I reread the pathology report, bilateral breast cancer. I looked up from the chart. "What other options? Maybe we can get her into St. Luke's access program?"

"That's what I was hoping. But you have to explain it to her. She doesn't speak English very well."

"Okay, then let's get her on the line and you translate for me..."

"There's more." Olga's dark eyes grew darker.

"More?" I said, dreading the answer.

"Her family doesn't know yet."

"What? They don't know she has breast cancer. She's had this for seven months and they don't know?"

Olga nodded and continued, "I told her I would help her fill out the paperwork, even go to the hospital with her. I explained that we had ways to help her; that's when she said she hasn't told her family yet."

I stared at her. "How could her family not know?"

"Remember her son was getting married and she didn't want to spoil his wedding?"

I nodded.

"Then her husband got laid off and it was around Christmas and she didn't want them to be upset. They got behind on bills. She kept trying to get approval at the clinic but when they turned her down, she gave up."

"She has to be worried," I said

"Oh, she is. She's terrified," Olga responded.

"Okay, you need to go get her and bring her here to talk to me," I said.

Olga spun around and was out the door, nearly running over Pam, whose grim face told me we had another problem.

"Can I see you a minute?"

"What's up?"

"I think we're going to have a problem with our new radiologist." Pam's hands were full of papers.

"Now what?" I sighed.

"Remember how she kept insisting that she wasn't worried about how much money she made? How she could work with us? She was happy to be here, happy to be able to help the poor?"

I nodded.

"Well, I think her definition of happiness has changed. She's asking me if we are going to advance her against what we think we will be collecting. I said we didn't usually do that. There's no provision for it in her contract, I checked. But I thought I better talk to you."

This radiologist had been with us only six weeks, and we had waited over two months for her to come on board. We had convinced ourselves she was worth it and made do with locum tenums to provide coverage.

Dixie had been so excited about this radiologist, thinking she was the answer to our prayers. She was a good radiologist with lots of experience, and she had told us that she really loved mammography—a rarity in itself. We had learned that most radiologists only get excited about MRIs, CAT scans, those procedures that guarantee high dollar reimbursement. Most wanted nothing to do with mammography. It was tedious work, the reimbursement was low, and the risk of lawsuits was exceptionally high. In fact, failure to diagnose breast cancer had become the number one cause of medical lawsuits in the United States.

This radiologist came from a public health setting. The positive thing for us was that she was accustomed to dealing with an uninsured population. The bad part was that she was used to being paid a guaranteed salary. We had talked at great lengths during our negotiations about reimbursement, outlining in detail how we paid against collections and the formula for compensating the sponsored procedures. Money was not an issue, she had assured us. She and her husband were well off. She wanted to have quality time with him, and she wanted out of the politics of the university. She had convinced us that she wanted to be part of The Rose for all the right reasons.

"I don't believe this, Pam," I said. A bad feeling was forming in my tummy. "We were so careful about explaining her reimbursement. I thought she understood. What would her check be this month?"

When Pam told me the amount, I knew it wasn't going to fly. My heart sank. We were going to have to pay ahead or look for another radiologist. I authorized an advance for $10,000. I knew we had almost that amount in receivables coming to us for the past month's work.

As Pam turned to leave, she said over her shoulder, "I will cut the check, but you'll need to give it to her. You'll need to explain how we came up with this amount. She wants to talk to you anyway."

"When will it be ready?"

"End of the day." Pam was gone.

"Okay," I murmured, thinking that the morning was shot. I left my office, walked across the hall to Verlyn's office, intent on reviewing the final section of the grant, when the intercom crackled overhead.

"Dorothy, please return to your office." There was no mistaking Olga's voice.

As I started back I made one detour, stopping at Pat's office. She was our accounting person and a survivor. I stuck my head in, and said, "Pat, I may need you in my office in a few minutes."

"No problem," she responded. "What for?"

"You may have to help me convince one of our sponsored patients that she needs to get treatment."

Pat nodded. No further explanation was needed.

When I entered my office, Olga introduced Ms. Gonzales. She was a short, neatly dressed woman of average size. She acknowledged me with a pleasant smile that immediately faded. She looked at Olga. As we sat down at my tiny conference table, she sat straight up, her back pushed against the chair, her knees held tightly together, feet flat on the floor. Her purse sat on her lap; she gripped it with both hands. Her face was unlined. There was a softness to her. She smelled of fresh bread. Her eyes were sharp and clear and filled with fear.

I looked into those eyes and, with Olga translating, got straight to the point.

Yes, she understood she had cancer. Yes, she had gone to the clinic and been turned away. Yes, she knew she must get treatment and understood that we were trying to help her. No, her family did not know yet. She looked down, studying her hands, refusing to meet my eyes any longer.

At this point, Pat came in. From the moment she joined us, the tension in the room deepened. We briefly explained to Pat what was going on and told Ms. Gonzales that Pat was a survivor, nearly three years out.

With Olga translating, Pat talked openly about her own experience with cancer and her treatment. Pat shared her fears. At one point, Pat said, "I think Ms. Gonzales understands what I am saying."

Ms. Gonzales responded, "I understand a little English but can't talk it much." She was stoic. No emotion registered on her face until Pat asked about her children.

"Do you have boys or girls?" Pat asked, leaning into the table. Her gaze was direct.

"Both," Ms. Gonzales responded, her voice still guarded.

"Tell me about your son," Pat said.

Ms. Gonzales lit up. She suddenly became animated and, in very broken English, described her son. He sounded quite the gentleman and was obviously her pride and joy.

"He loves you a lot, doesn't he?" Pat smiled, "And you love him."

Ms. Gonzales nodded.

Pat reached across the table, touched Ms. Gonzales's hand, and said softly, "Your children need to know, especially your son. He would want to know. He would want to do whatever he could to help his Mama get well."

Ms. Gonzales's shoulders slumped. She sighed. Tears filled her eyes. She looked down and nodded.

Pat touched her hand again. "You can call me anytime," Pat encouraged as she stood up to leave. The tension in the room evaporated. The ground was level again, and we talked about what was ahead for her and what had to happen for her to get treatment. I assured her Olga could accompany her to any of the appointments if needed.

She sent a grateful look to Olga. They left together to return to Ms. Gonzales's home.

Even then, I realized that hospitals would probably have handled this situation very differently, but we weren't a hospital and we didn't have social services. We did have employees who cared and we used what we had at hand to do what we needed to do.

Feeling better, thinking something had actually been accomplished this day, I set out in search of Verlyn and our $100,000 proposal. An hour ago it was nowhere near finished. She wasn't in her office. Betting that she had gone to lunch, I fumed all the way to the front office, when I heard her voice.

She was standing by the copy machine. It was open and its innards were lying around. The repairman was saying he'd never seen such a mess and Verlyn was literally hopping up and down, badgering him about how long it would take to fix it.

"I only needed one more copy out of it!" she wailed. "We have to send eight copies of this proposal! Today! It's fifty pages long. Every time I try to work with this machine it breaks down. I swear it doesn't like me. Can't you do anything?" she pleaded with him, clutching his arm, her voice near hysteria. I was sure the repairman just wished this crazy lady would go away.

"Verlyn, calm down. Take it to Office Depot..."

Before the words got out of my mouth, the repairman snapped the cover closed with a "It's ready!"

"Thank goodness!" Verlyn exclaimed, nearly jumping over the man to get to the machine. She laughed; her smile froze when she saw the look on my face. I wasn't finding any of this very funny.

"Oh, Dorothy, don't worry so. It will be fine. I'll send it Federal Express. I would have gotten in the car and driven it to San Antonio if I had to."

"It's supposed to be going to Austin, Verlyn," I groaned, scouring the pages, searching for the address.

"Oh! I meant Austin," she sighed, her flitting around disappeared and she was all business. Even so, I insisted on seeing the Fed Ex shipping label to be sure it was clearly marked to Austin.

My head had started to ache. It was about 2 o'clock. I wandered back to my office. Olga had returned.

"How did it go?" I asked her.

She started reporting with her customary no-nonsense professionalism, sharing only the important facts.

When they had returned to Ms. Gonzales's house, oddly enough the husband and two of the children were there, including the son. Olga had stayed while Ms. Gonzales explained what had been happening. Olga said, "I sat in another room while she told her family. When she finished, I talked with all of them."

In Olga's opinion, they understood the importance of getting her into treatment. They were upset to hear the news but they seemed supportive. Olga's report continued as she told me that she had called St. Luke's and Ms. Gonzales would be seen on Friday.

I was about to ask her if we needed to provide transportation when the radiologist walked into my office and announced that she needed to talk to me. Before I answered, Olga was gone. I put on my brightest face and invited the doctor to sit down. It didn't take long to size up the lay of the land.

She advised me that even with the advance against collections, it wasn't enough. Without any preliminaries, she said she was quitting and in fact already had a position with a local hospital. She would give us the required sixty days but wondered if we could wind things up before then.

My head was spinning. I weighed our options, of which there were none. We needed to find another radiologist and find one pretty damn quickly. She asked me again about releasing her early from the contract, adding that it would really make her happy if we could do that.

At that moment, her happiness was not one of my priorities.

She left my office. I walked out behind her, intending to go to Pam's office for the radiologist's check. Instead, something steered me back through the maze of halls to Olga's area.

Olga was sitting at her desk, staring straight ahead, her eyes were glazed.

"Olga, are you all right?" I asked

Startled, she looked up. Her eyes still unfocused, an unusual stillness surrounded her. "Dorothy, you know about that thing, it's like coincidence, I think the word in English is serendipity?"

I nodded.

"Something very strange happened at Ms. Gonzales's house. The reason I didn't call you from there was they cut off her phone. I had finished the call to St. Luke's. I hung up and when I picked it up to call you, the phone was dead. Isn't it strange how there was just enough time to make that phone call to St. Luke's?"

"They cut off her phone? What do you mean?" I panicked.

"They are three months behind on all their bills; they will probably lose their home too. Remember, he had been out of work. They don't have any money."

"Olga, listen to me," I said sharply. Her eyes widened. I knew Olga was having a tough time coping with the events of the afternoon, but she didn't realize the impact of the phone being disconnected. If we couldn't reach Ms. Gonzales, we would be back to square one.

"Please," I said more gently, "Call Southwestern Bell. Find me someone to talk to, we must convince them to turn that phone back on, at least for another couple of weeks. I know they can do that. We have to be able to reach her. She has to have a phone. Call me when you get through to a supervisor. I've got to see Pam, but then I'll be back in my office.

Olga was reaching for the phone book as I started to turn to leave. I stopped and said, "Are you okay? Olga?"

Tears glistened in her eyes but her voice was matter of fact. "Do you know why they turned her down at the clinic?" She paused and looked at me before continuing, "She didn't have any idea how much money her husband made. He had never told her and she wouldn't ask. Even when he was working full time, she didn't know. It's one of those things. The men don't always tell their wives what they make.

When the clinic insisted she provide proof of income, she was afraid to ask, she gave up."

My heart sank. Six months wasted.

The voice over the intercom announced that Dixie was returning my call on line two.

I dreaded having to tell her the news about the radiologist. Dixie was astonished. To every "But she told us..." I would respond with "I know, Dixie, that's what she told us." Dixie closed our discussion by saying that this radiologist just "wasn't the right one." She was trying to make me feel better. It didn't work.

As I hung up, Olga stuck her head in the door.

"I talked to a supervisor."

"You did? Really?"

The look on her face was serious. "I figured I would try to talk to them first and then if they said no, I would get you."

"And?"

"They are going to leave the phone on." Her smile lit up the room.

"Good work, Olga," I exclaimed—resisting jumping up and giving her a hug—that wasn't her style or mine, then.

She left as Pam walked in, waving the check at me.

"I still don't understand. I can't believe this is happening," I said as I signed the check. "Dixie and I were so clear about the work, the amount of pay, everything. She was the one who wanted to work with poor people, wanted a less stressful job. I can't believe we're looking again. I wish I knew what we were doing wrong." I looked up at Pam, pleading, "Tell me Pam, what is going on?"

Pam looked at me, sighed and leaned against the door jam. Her eyes softened. "Dorothy, it's always a matter of money."

I returned her gaze. Picking up my briefcase and walking to the door, I flipped the light switch to off.

"You're right, Pam. For The Rose...for our patients...it's always a matter of money."

Chapter 13
Go Find a Doctor

The call came about 2 o'clock in the afternoon.

"I don't know if I have the right place or not," a female voice said, "but the American Cancer Society told me to call you."

"Yes?" I replied.

"This is The Rose, is that right? The lady who answered your phone said I needed to talk to you. I was afraid I had gotten cut off when she transferred me to you. This is the tenth call I've made to different places trying to find some help. I'm at a pay phone and I don't have many more quarters left. So I hope you're the one I need to talk to." Her words tumbled out.

"I probably am. Tell me what's going on."

She began her story.

"My name is Jerri and I'm 36 years old," she said. "I found a lump in my breast about four months ago. I was hoping it would go away but it didn't, so I finally got a mammogram at the diagnostic center downtown. I heard that was what I needed to do, get a mammogram, but it cost $125 so I had to wait till payday. Then they said I needed an ultrasound and that was another $250. Then they said I needed to see a surgeon, and so I did and he said I had cancer and I would need surgery. First he had to do a biopsy, and that was going to be another $1,000, and then when I had it done, it was for sure that I had cancer." She paused. "We don't have any insurance."

I remember thinking that in spite of having breast cancer, this woman was oddly calm. Of course, she'd repeated this story ten times during the past couple of hours, so maybe she was on automatic pilot. It was much later when I learned of her terror.

She continued to chronicle the last few weeks. "The surgeon said he would work with us for his cost, we could pay him out, but I would have to go to the hospital to have a mastectomy and I needed to have it done pretty quickly. My husband is a mechanic and makes $9 an hour, we have about $350 every two weeks to work with, but our car is broken right now. We don't have much money. I went to the hospital and talked to the people about making payments. They wanted a credit card, but we don't have one. We always pay our own way. I have a nine-year-old son and the last time I was in the hospital was when I had him. Anyway, the hospital said that we could pay it out but they needed $1,250 as a down payment. So we called our relatives and finally my husband's uncle loaned us the money. Then when I got to the hospital they wouldn't let me have the surgery until they had another $750 down payment for the anesthesiology. My husband was frantic and started making more calls. Finally another relative put it on a credit card."

By now, I was enthralled with this woman's story. I kept trying to figure out why she had called us; she had already had a mammogram, an ultrasound, and a biopsy. Those were the services I could have offered her. Maybe she was looking for a support group or information on reconstruction. I waited, listening. Her words were halting; she had a childlike manner of speaking.

"So I had the mastectomy. That was a week ago and today I went back to see the surgeon. He said the cancer was real bad. Something about the pathology report."

"Did you see that report?" I interrupted.

"Yes," she said, "I can read it to you."

Before I could stop her, she had put the phone down and I heard her fumbling with papers. The sounds of traffic filled the space, horns honking, the starting and stopping of engines. When she returned, she immediately launched into reading the report, stumbling over some of the words, sounding them out. She was right, the cancer was bad.

When she finished, I simply said, "Okay," and asked, "Then what happened?"

She continued, "The surgeon said I would need to have chemotherapy and I needed it right away. I thought the surgery was all I would need, I thought that was it. No one ever said anything about chemotherapy." She paused.

"Yes, Jerri," I said, filling up the silence, "chemotherapy sounds like the right course of treatment."

"He arranged for me to go see an onconologist—is that what they are called?" she asked.

"Oncologist," I responded, automatically correcting her pronunciation of the term.

"The oncologist," she said the word perfectly, "his office was just down the hall from the surgeon's office, so the surgeon called him to arrange for me to go right over. The surgeon said I shouldn't wait, I needed to go right then."

I was growing uncomfortable now, the small knot forming in my stomach was sending out loud signals. Jerri had stopped talking again, I was afraid we had gotten cut off.

Finally, I heard a deep inhale and she continued, "I was in his office, the oncologist. I had taken my chart with me and he was sitting behind his desk and looking over it. He said, 'Yes, this is very serious, and we have to start chemotherapy immediately.' I asked when. He said he would schedule the first treatment this Thursday and then I would need six to nine more every three to four weeks. 'How much is this going to cost?' I asked him. He said, 'Cost?' I said, 'Yes, I will have to find the money because we don't have insurance.' He said it was very expensive, thousands of dollars."

Now Jerri's voice broke. I waited.

"Then he handed my chart back to me and he said, 'Go find another doctor. I can't help you.'" Her voice cracked again.

Another pause, finally, in my softest voice, I asked, "He handed your chart back to you?"

She said, "Yes." She didn't remember what else was said, she was so upset. She just remembered thanking him and taking her chart. She left the office, walked outside, found the nearest pay phone and looked up hospitals listed in the yellow pages and started calling them. "I was lucky there was a book here in the phone booth," she said.

Lucky? I thought.

She continued, "I called a lot of places, five or six hospitals, when finally someone said to call Reach to Recovery at the American Cancer Society and they were the ones that said to call The Rose."

My mind was reeling. I knew there had to be a way to help her, but first things first.

"Jerri, let's start over. Do you have a phone at home?"

"We used to, but it's been disconnected."

"And your surgery was a week ago?"

"Yes, I still have the drains in."

I almost lost it then. It was hot outside. Houston can be hot any time of year, but this week in November was miserably hot. I imagined the scene at the other end of the phone line: a young woman standing at a pay phone, fighting off the heat and the fumes from the downtown traffic, feeding one coin after another into a pay phone, hoping against hope to find help, with her drains still in place, protruding out from under her skin.

"Jerri, you are talking to Dorothy, don't forget this name. Give me the phone number on that pay phone please."

There was a pause and she said, "I don't see one. It's not on here."

"Okay, then is your husband with you?"

"No, I took the bus; he had to work today. He's already missed too much on account of me and we need the money. I lost my job when I got sick, it was only a part-time job but it was something. They didn't need me anymore. We don't have much money now."

"Can you give me his work phone number?" I asked.

"I don't know it; I never call him there."

"Where does he work?" Again, I prodded. I could tell she was uncomfortable, she hesitated, maybe worried I would call him and he'd lose his job, so I changed my approach.

"Jerri, we will find you help but let me explain some things. We don't do chemotherapy here at The Rose, but I will find someone who does and who can help you." *I hope*, I said silently to myself. "I want to be sure I have a way to reach you, just in case something happens and we get cut off during this phone call."

She understood and gave me his name and where he worked.

"Are you feeling well enough to stay on the line for a little while longer?" I asked.

She said, "Yes, I just have to be home when my son gets out of school, around 4:30."

I was so incredulous I almost laughed. Her priorities were absolutely clear. She had to be home for her son by 4:30.

I, on the other hand, had started to panic, mentally weighing the best approach and whom to call to try to get her into the public health system. Most of all, I knew I couldn't let her hang up because I had such a bad feeling that I'd never find her again.

So I said, "No matter what, Jerri, stay on this line. I'm going to put you on hold and make some calls. Do not hang up. Promise me that."

She said okay, then she asked me, "Who are you again?"

I said, "Dorothy Weston."

She asked, "I mean, what do you do at The Rose, what is your job? I could call you back. I've already taken up so much of your time. Are you sure it's okay for you to keep talking to me?"

I said, "It's okay, Jerri. I'm the boss."

That was the moment she broke down and cried. For the next four or five minutes, she cried, big sobs pouring out between her words of "I'm sorry", "I'm so sorry." She cried. I talked, telling her it would be all right. She cried some more, I kept talking.

By now I had caught the attention of one of the employees who was passing by my office, frantically I motioned for her to come into the room. While reassuring Jerri, I had found the numbers needed from my Rolodex, so I scribbled notes to my employee, asking her to start making the phone calls.

I glanced at my watch, 2:50 p.m. I had been on the phone for nearly an hour. It was a Friday afternoon, so finding someone still in their office would be a trick.

My employee returned, indicating some success.

I said to Jerri, "I want you to talk with one of my employees now, while I talk to a couple of people."

Within the next hour, we made a dozen phone calls. I knew that we had already tapped out our local oncologist. Next were calls to the county hospital district and frustrating minutes of being kept on hold with the eligibility office. Then a call to the clinic assigned to her zip code. The public health folks kept saying that she needed to come in for a consultation and to have an initial screening.

"She already has breast cancer!" I almost screamed into the telephone. I gave up and went another way.

Finally, I reached Dr. Nancy Neff at Ben Taub Hospital and she intervened. Between about six people and as many phone calls, everything was set up. Jerri's application for public health would be expedited and her chemotherapy started the following week.

It took a while for Jerri to understand what we were doing. She had never accepted charity before, had always paid her own way. It took some time to convince her that she wasn't going to have to get another loan from anyone. She didn't understand that she could qualify for public health. I was asking a lot of questions about her finances and demographics and work history so she could be assigned to the right referring clinic, and she was suspicious of the whole process.

Her doctor would take the drains out on Wednesday morning; her chemotherapy consult at Ben Taub would be that same afternoon. We had reached her doctor and explained the situation. He had no clue about the outcome of Jerri's visit with the oncologist.

Of course, Jerri had a few other worries, such as having grocery money for the week. They had used every penny from their savings for the diagnostic work-up and biopsy. My heart dropped when she told me that because we could have helped her there—had she known about us.

Our employees got together and provided Jerri's family with Thanksgiving dinner. She started her chemotherapy. We received a couple of letters from her, but the last one sounded as if more hard times had hit that family. We lost track of her.

Jerri's plight haunted me. Her story was the example Verlyn used in the introduction of an ambitious grant proposal to St. Luke's Episcopal Health Charities.

"Go find a doctor" were the first words of the proposal, then we described the scene of the oncologist handing Jerri back her chart.

We needed "a better way," the proposal explained. The community needed The Rose to do more than provide mammograms and biopsies. What we needed was a physician network and a staff assigned to navigate women through the system. It wouldn't happen overnight, but we needed the seed funding to start.

The Charities agreed and their grant award launched the patient navigation program that is now modeled throughout the nation.

Jerri left a legacy for The Rose that was uniquely her own.

Post script: On 12-15-2003, I received a note, handwritten in gold ink on a small Christmas card that said:

I just like to say Thank You so very very much—it has been five years now but I don't know if it would have—if not for you all!
May God Bless you All!
Merry Christmas from Jerri & family

Chapter 14
Navigating New Waters

We approached 1998 battered but encouraged because we had recruited a group of radiologists who agreed to provide regular part-time on-site coverage. It would be years before we finally found radiologists who could provide full-time coverage, but at least now we could actually plan ahead and create a workflow.

It was during that same time period that the Episcopal Health Charities provided a three-year grant to establish a real patient navigation program. As much sense as it makes today, that wasn't the case then. I'd never heard of a program like the one I envisioned.

The experiences with Jerri and Ms. Gonzales made it clear that our women did not need another frigging brochure explaining the procedures or what they were about to go through. What they needed was a real live person by their side. That person had to be street savvy, able to understand the culture of the person they were helping, and know how to find those 'back doors' to care. That person had to communicate with the patients in their own language and know when the patient did not comprehend what she heard, even if the words were in a language she understood. Most of all, our patient navigator had to be willing to walk alongside each woman through her journey, even when there was nothing else that could be done to help her.

It was no small task to navigate someone through the maze of traditional medicine, through the medical jargon and through the days of treatment. No small task to be another person's compass when they got off track or were too afraid to take another step.

Years later, hospitals would implement patient navigation programs for different reasons. It was a way to keep the business within their four walls and not have their patients go to the medical center or specialty hospital across the street. I'm not saying women in those hospitals didn't benefit from having a navigator, of course they did. But the hospital's programs served only insured patients. Nobody had programs for the uninsured.

Our patient navigation program had an added challenge: The Rose wasn't a hospital. We didn't have four walls to keep women 'in.' We had to convince hospitals and doctors and clinics and radiation therapy centers and surgery centers and infusion centers and laboratories to work with us and provide treatment. I had figured out early on that we also had to build a physician network if we wanted to have anywhere to 'navigate' our uninsured women to when they needed treatment.

"Help us take care of only one woman a year," I bargained, strong in my conviction that one woman's life was not a lot to ask for. "I promise your office staff won't have to handle anything. Our navigators will make sure the patient has had the lab and x-ray pre-surgery tests, we'll find an anesthesiologist and the outpatient surgery center, and we'll handle moving her into chemotherapy with an oncologist." Just one woman, that's all we asked for, but our pleas fell on deaf ears—at first.

The docs complained that they were already giving away too much care with the lousy reimbursement from insurance companies. The medical facilities said they weren't in the business of caring for the uninsured. Taking care of 'those kinds of people' was the responsibility of the public health hospitals and the reason we paid so much in taxes!

We had hired Janet Hoagland, MD, to be the director of the physician network program and she tried her best but couldn't convince her colleagues to help. Yet having Janet on board was a blessing and her coming to The Rose was another miracle.

She had faced and won her own battle with cancer. As a well-respected and sought after breast surgeon, her services were in high demand, but fighting for her life became her only priority, which meant closing her office. Five years later, recovered and healthy, she was ready to return to work but not as a general surgeon.

Janet provided the physician coverage we needed at the second location, doing ultrasounds and biopsies and patient counseling. Someone else would have to build the physician network; Janet soon became irreplaceable as a physician to our patients. We received hundreds of letters exhorting her kindness and I often wondered if our patients, especially our uninsured patients, ever realized that they were receiving care from one of the leading breast surgeons in the city.

She was a physician who really cared—I cannot list the number of times she went to bat for our women, fighting the Medical Center bureaucrats, arguing that an uninsured woman should receive "the same level of care as an insured woman would!"

Our first two patient navigators were amazing women. Monica

was new to The Rose and had a strong personality that almost intimidated most folks. Cris, who was a little softer in her approach but every bit as strong, had worked her way up through the ranks of The Rose. Both knew their stuff, cared, and were among the first navigators to be certified in the state.

About the time the navigators were up to speed, we found the right person in Sharon to sell our concept of a volunteer physician network. Sharon could sell anyone most anything, but I'm convinced it was the homemade cookies she carried to the physicians' offices that sealed the deal. Before long, she had testimonies from other doctors in our physician network, praising our navigators and saying all they had to do whenever they had an uninsured woman who needed service was call The Rose. That was the key selling point.

At some point every physician encounters a patient who isn't insured; most often she is someone they have cared for before who has lost her insurance. When Sharon called on new physicians and they finally understood the value of the program and how it could help patients in their own practice, they couldn't sign up fast enough. By the end of the three-year grant, Sharon had recruited over 400 physicians.

Usually the surgeons would provide mastectomies pro-bono and convinced their hospitals to do the same. It was wonderful having so many champions on our side. Thank goodness there was funding from Susan G. Komen-Houston. We created a treatment fund, mainly to pay a pre-agreed portion of the cost of chemotherapy to the oncologists and to offset other clinical costs. Somehow our navigators managed to move one uninsured woman after another into treatment. Every case was reviewed, every woman needed different services, but somehow the program worked.

Every time I thought we couldn't expand or add different services, our patients would show us the need. When we began diagnosing more women who were under forty years old, Janet and Amy started the Knockout Roses. It was the first breast cancer support group totally geared for young women. Janet was someone who had 'been there,' she could talk their talk, was intimate with their fears, and understood exactly what they meant when they shared their worries about seeing their children grow up.

Another support group that emerged during that time was Las Rosas Vivas. Not long after Ms. Gonzales finished her treatment, she convinced us that we needed a support group for women who spoke Spanish, and she became one of its founding members.

Five support groups met each month within our walls—the Rose Garden had been going strong since 1987, The Rosebuds started at the second center in 1992, next came the Rosebuds 2 for women dealing with reoccurrence and metastatic breast cancer and issues that were different than a woman diagnosed for the first time. Together with the Hispanic group and the young women's group, those groups meant lots of meetings and lots of support.

We were muddling along at The Rose. It was a difficult year for fundraising, but for me nothing compared to the difficulty happening on the home front. Unfortunately, things there had gone from bad to worse.

Chapter 15
The Final Straw

My Saucy dog was dying and cancer had invaded my life in a different way.

The walks with Saucy every evening had become the highlight of my day. She would literally bounce up and down waiting for me to put my shoes on and connect her leash. Hooked up, it was a race out the door and down the sidewalk with her pulling so fast I could barely keep up; at least until the day came when she could only manage a block or so before she had to stop. There was no moving Saucy once she sat down. She would pant heavily and look away, as if embarrassed. At first I thought she was just getting older, nine years is old for a dog as big as Saucy.

Then I found the growth behind her ear. The vet confirmed it was cancer.

Not everyone would opt for chemotherapy for a pet, but we did. Alan took her in for the first consult and, listening to him later, I was actually encouraged. The cost was steep, $3,000, but as he understood it she had a good chance if she stayed on chemo for at least nine months. Over the months ahead, Saucy became more active and I cherished seeing her run again. It was almost like having a puppy. I had no idea of the level of pain she must have endured prior to the chemo.

Within a month of ending chemotherapy, the tumor was back. I was shocked! Sure, I knew cancers return, but so quickly? For whatever reason, I had never considered that possibility.

This time I was the one who took her to the vet, and she explained that she had told my husband that as long as Saucy stayed on chemotherapy it might keep the cancer at bay but it would not eliminate it.

"He heard what he wanted to hear," she said gently, "obviously Saucy means a lot to both of you." She had no idea how true that was. Caring for Saucy had kept us living in the same house together; our marriage had been over a long time ago. This creature, who long ago had won over Alan's heart, was the single common thread we still shared in life.

The vet continued, "I never gave her more than a year to live. I told him that when he first brought her in." She said she had been surprised that we decided to have the treatment and she was also surprised at the cancer's aggressiveness upon its return. "She might respond to another round of chemotherapy, but you would only be buying a little more time."

A little more time was all I wanted, and what I dreaded the most. No, I wouldn't put her through chemotherapy again, or make us walk through that senseless valley of hope against hope.

Each day the tumor grew and each day I pushed away thoughts of the inevitable. Selfishly, I prayed that she would die on her own and spare me from having to make that final decision. She didn't move around much, didn't eat much. The tumor soon encompassed most of her massive neck.

It was three weeks after the chemotherapy ended, a Sunday afternoon, and Saucy lay on the rug near the back door. She was watching me as I sat on the couch. Those brown black eyes were filled with pain, yet there was something else. It was the same look she had had with Mary Louise, the same knowing that death was near.

"Tomorrow, Saucy. We'll do it tomorrow," I promised.

I stretched out on the rug beside her. With my arms around her, I buried my face in her fur, breathing in the scent that was Saucy's alone. My thoughts tried to go to 'this time tomorrow' but I could not imagine life without her.

The next day she lay on the vet's exam table. I stood behind her, stroking her back, touching every part of her, trying to memorize the feel of her. We were in a special room, one I had never been in before, far to the back side of the clinic. As we waited, I realized this room had an exit door to the outside. A chill ran over me, we would be able to leave without having to go back through the main area, without having to see all the other pets and their owners. We would leave with Saucy's body but not with her.

"Are we ready?" the vet asked, holding up the syringe that would end her life. I nodded.

Alan took my arm and gently moved me around to the front of the table. "Stand here," he said, "so the last thing she sees will be you."

The moment Saucy's eyes met mine the theme song from *Titanic* started playing over the speakers. "Near, Far, wherever you are...My heart will go on." The words pierced through me. *Maybe someday,* I thought, *but not now.* That day, my heart wanted to stop with hers. I held back my sobs until she closed her eyes.

Saucy dog died on July 1, 1998, and whatever bond Alan and I had shared was gone with her. Finding a way to end a long-time marriage was like trying to get rid of sticker burrs that cling to your socks after a walk in the woods. It hurts to pull them out, but it hurts more to leave them in.

During that same year of Saucy's bout with cancer, I learned my younger brother, Jerry, was terminally ill. He and I had a strange relationship, sometimes we were close, sometimes not, but he was the one person who could always make me laugh. I made a lot of day trips to Nacogdoches to see him. The trip was long, four hours up and four hours back. I really couldn't afford a motel to stay overnight. It had been a long time between jobs for Alan. But those four hours gave me plenty of time to think. I always made those trips alone.

I had hit rock bottom, heartsick from all the death around me. We were also hitting rock bottom at work.

It was December of 1998, during those hypnotically mind-numbing weeks between Thanksgiving and Christmas when folks work by rote, their thoughts consumed with Holiday planning.

"We have only $25,000 left in the bank." Pam's voice shook as she laid the paper in front of me.

"What does that mean exactly?" I asked.

"If something doesn't come in this week, we won't be able to make payroll," she whispered. Her face was flushed and her breathing had stopped—snatched away by the fear that had come alive in the room.

"It will come," I said calmly.

"Have you called Komen?" she asked. "Maybe if you told them what was happening…"

The look on my face stopped her. I wasn't calling Komen. In their granting process, they had moved their award dates from October to later in the year. It could be January or February of the next year before we knew IF we had received funding and how much had been granted. Calling them when the grant may not have even been approved was not an option in my book.

"Is there anything else coming in?" she said. Her voice was husky, hope danced around her question. Pam was not given to public displays of emotion, but today she was on the edge of a complete meltdown. Her wide-set eyes bored into me.

"Don't you realize, even if we found money for this payroll, there won't be any left for the next one?" her voice rose a couple of octaves higher. She shook her head, "I can't believe I let us get to this point, I should have been paying more attention…"

"No, not in grants," I said, stopping her. "Is there anything else we can delay paying?"

We spent a few minutes reviewing the list of bills owed. What few bills we had could wait for another month. Payroll could not.

I got up and walked around the desk, patting her on the arm. "It will come, Pam," I said quietly. "I just know it will."

Actually, I didn't know for sure but I was conjuring up a plan. I would withdraw my retirement funds. It wasn't a lot of money, but would get us through a couple of months. It was the only retirement I had, earned while working at Bayshore.

My other solution was a short-term loan from Louise, the grant writer who used to work for us. When her husband died, she was left with a nice inheritance. She had moved away but kept in touch. When I called her explaining the amount we needed to cover payroll, she was so gracious, immediately agreeing to send it. She added that we could pay it back whenever our next big grant came in. But days passed and the check didn't arrive.

The last part of my plan was to keep calling on St. Theresa of the little flower. And sure enough, every day a rose appeared, on a card, as a gift, in a bud vase, so I stood firm in my faith that something would happen—something good.

Even so, the next few days were pure hell.

Three days before payroll, Louise's check arrived. It got us through the first payday in December. I was so grateful.

Between that payroll and Christmas, the Komen award arrived in the mail. We could breathe again.

Years later, Pam told that story during a staff meeting and I was genuinely surprised to see the tears running down her face. "I don't know how Dorothy knew we'd get through that time," she said. "She kept telling me the money would come. I couldn't get over her absolute belief."

Belief? True. Absolute? Maybe, but only because of the back-up plan.

But I didn't have a back-up plan for my personal life. The weekend trips to see my brother left me frazzled and sad; seeing Jerry's health fade more each time I visited was grueling. The tension at home worsened. Yet work continued to consume me and maybe even console me. I wrote more grants, and little by little, we pulled ahead of the curve at The Rose. The months flew by and suddenly another year had passed.

On January 25, 2000, Jerry died. The death certificate showed the cause as cirrhosis of the liver. But I knew he died of a broken spirit after his marriage ended years earlier and he couldn't find work. I also knew it hadn't taken long before alcohol was his only companion. I had started to become familiar with that feeling; I worried that I was drinking too much, using it to assuage my own spirit that was battered at every turn.

The stress of another year of scraping by at home and at work was showing on me. I was tired of being resentful every time I came home to someone who didn't work, knowing the bills were piling up. I was tired of trying to pretend all was well with my friends and church family.

Mainly I was tired of the daily debate I had with myself about calling the marriage quits. *After twenty years with this man,* I argued, *I can't just give up.* I reminded myself that some of those years had been good ones. We had been comfortable with each other and he had always been supportive of The Rose, never criticizing the long hours I spent at work, always willing to be the perfect escort to functions. In any marriage, it takes two, to make it and to end it.

It seemed like I was fighting some kind of battle, internal or external, all the time. Painful, take-your-breath-away painful, breakouts of shingles had become a routine occurrence—always appearing after some crisis.

I struggled with big welts traveling up and down my arms, made more red and irritated by the scratching. "Nerves," the doctor pronounced. "You need to find a way to handle your stress level." That was easier said than done.

On the Sunday my sisters and I buried my brother Jerry, I returned home, walked into the kitchen and found Alan reading the paper. I could barely think; my eyes were swollen from crying during the entire four-hour trip back home. Grief burst from every cell of my being.

It had been a sad little funeral, my brother's body was too yellow to allow a viewing and his young son could barely manage the cost of having him buried in a real cemetery. I didn't have an extra penny to give him.

I looked at the man I'd shared space with for twenty years and asked for a divorce. It was final sixty days later.

Chapter 16
Buildings, Beloved, and Believing Again

It was June, 2001. The feasibility study for our proposed $10 million capital campaign had just been completed and according to Maria, our campaign counsel, it was a Stellar Study.

The Rose had a Stellar reputation and our campaign should have Stellar results. Maria loved using the word 'stellar' but she was pretty impressed with her findings—and so were we.

She had visited with 28 foundations, testing the waters, asking if they would support a capital campaign for us to buy a building and all the equipment needed to have a first class center. Each of them agreed that after fifteen years of service The Rose needed to have a home of its own.

We were leasing space in a building we had been in since the early '90s and were bursting at the seams. First we considered a piece of property to build on, but at the magical deciding moment the owner of the building we occupied started making noises that he'd like to sell it. He would even carry the down payment while we raised the rest. I was so excited.

Of course, that year I was excited for a lot of reasons, and for the first time in nearly two decades that excitement had nothing to do with The Rose. I had met someone special and was enjoying the romance of a lifetime.

It all started one Wednesday night while I was on the internet at home. Most folks forget how novel the internet was in the early 2000s. It was almost a luxury to have such a modern communications system at work or at home, even if it was slower than slow and you had to mess with modems and wait for dial-ups to go through.

Plenty of companies were struggling with how much or how little the internet should be used. Even though we had internet at work, there were too many unknowns. I never trusted that the firewall was strong enough to protect our patient files. So, to be safe, I did most of my research for grants from home. Checking for new grant leads and reading articles about breast cancer had become a regular evening routine.

I had finished a short e-talk with my son on an instant messaging service called ICQ. The initials stood for Instant Chat Query and it was not well known or used much in the US. Instant messaging was in its infancy and there wasn't such a thing as Skype or FaceTime, none of the methods we use so easily today were available or even created yet.

But ICQ was standard in blue collar communities and a major messaging service for other countries, especially Canada. My son knew about it because he was in a locksmith's online forum. Before I e-talked with him, I had also chatted with an Australian breast cancer support group using ICQ.

I sat staring at the screen, it was late and the silence in the house screamed from every corner. Friends and colleagues had told me that the modern way to meet people was through the internet. After all, I was fifty years old and going to bars to meet someone was not an option.

There wasn't a single eligible man at church, and for some odd reason all my 'friends' kept saying they didn't know anyone 'good enough' for me. My friend Louise had recently moved to New York to start a new life with her true love, a great guy she had met online. She kept urging me to find a chat room, but I was too proud to admit that I didn't have a clue what that meant or how to get into one.

Maybe it was the glass of wine, maybe just the loneliness of all those empty years, whatever it was I found the chat section on ICQ and before I could stop myself I hit the send button after typing the words, "Do you want to dance and tell me your dreams?"

Little did I realize that request went to about a million people. Thank goodness only 35 responded—some were really strange, which I quickly eliminated, in fact I deleted all of them except one.

For the next eighteen months, this guy named Pat and I chatted occasionally. In the beginning he was just someone to talk to. I figured out pretty quickly that he didn't meet my criteria. I had these 'rules.' One was that I wasn't going to date anyone who lived more than forty miles away. Since he lived in Edmonton, Canada, he was never going to be a candidate.

I never thought of him as a love interest anyway. His children were so much younger than mine (I had David right out of high school) that I figured Pat had to be years younger than me, violating another one of my rules: no dating younger men. What on earth would I have in common with someone fifteen years younger than me? As it turned out, we were about the same age.

What I liked the most about e-talking with Pat was the way his mind worked. He could be irreverent one moment, thoughtful the next. He knew about so many different things that I wondered if he wasn't looking up information on the internet as we talked. Later on, I would learn that he has a great mind and also an uncanny memory about most topics, from the trivial to significant. We talked about everything, books, religion, politics and world issues. I could be myself and not worry about voicing my opinions. For the first five or six months, I didn't know if he was white, black or green, rich, poor or in between. It didn't matter, he was fun to talk to, and I started looking forward to chatting in the evenings.

After a few months, I did start seeing men through a dating service. After every date I'd go home, hoping to find Patrick online. When he was, I would tell him, "That guy didn't make it to first base!" or "What a jerk." And he'd say, "Oh? Tell me why?" And I'd blab everything the guy did or didn't do right. Believe me, if I had ever thought for one minute that I would end up with this Canadian, I wouldn't have told him squat.

As the months went by, he shared that working overseas was a lifelong goal and with his son finishing high school, the son who had lived with him following his divorce twelve years ago, he was applying for different international positions. One job looked promising and I encouraged him to go for it. I am such a believer in setting goals, I make at least 104 of my own each year and I love more than anything watching them materialize, so I urged him on.

A few weeks later, the deal was made, his contract signed. He was selling his home and preparing to leave for Abu Dhabi for two years. I was glad for him and said we had to keep emailing each other.

During an email exchange one evening, he typed, "I don't leave until June 13, and I have a friend in Houston [he didn't] that I am thinking about visiting." The message continued with "Is there any way you could get an extra day off during the Memorial Weekend and maybe we could meet for coffee or something? I could find a place to stay, a hotel somewhere convenient to you."

Even at this point, he didn't know I was a CEO of a company. I had learned early on that telling a guy my position ended up with him trying to find some way to take advantage of it or being intimidated by it. Whatever the reason, the knowledge seemed to change even the most promising relationship.

What Pat did know was that I wrote grants for a non-profit breast cancer organization. This was during that brief time in internet history before everything there was to know about a person was spread all over Google. I chuckled to myself and answered, "Sure, I'll try. Maybe

I can take an extra day off that weekend."

That email exchange occurred on May 4, 2001. During the next three weeks, our conversations changed, became flirty. By May 24, I had fallen so in love I could hardly stand it. Instead of him finding a hotel, I insisted he stay in my guest room. I wasn't worried; it wasn't like I was going to be alone with him. After all, my Episcopal priest (who was separated from his spouse) rented the mother-in-law apartment of my home. Besides, after fourteen months of talking, Patrick wasn't exactly a perfect stranger.

During one of the last email exchanges, I also offered to pick him up at the airport. That was when we finally exchanged photographs, which was a bit of a fiasco in itself, with mine never quite getting to him.

The most endearing message of that time was when I asked him, "How will I find you?" and he replied, "Look for someone wearing a café latte colored shirt, khaki pants…and a smile." From the moment I first saw that smile in person I was smitten.

The story of finding my beloved, the months that led up to finally meeting him, the ritual that I performed every Friday that brought him into my life, is a story for another book. But without a doubt, the joy his love brought gave me permission to find a new meaning in life. It was a good thing because life was about to become anything but joy-filled.

Four days after he left Houston, on June 6, I was on a plane to Canada to meet his family and to help him close up his home before he journeyed halfway around the world. When we said goodbye, I had no idea it would be nine months before we saw each other again.

While I was in Canada, a storm hit Houston, Tropical Storm Allison. It would drop 24 inches of rain on Houston in as many hours, flood the Medical Center, and end up causing billions of dollars in damage. I didn't know it then, but this tropical storm would ultimately be the first factor to cause the demise of our capital campaign.

In August, Maria presented her plan to the board, outlining all the steps needed to move forward with launching the capital campaign, the number of grants that would need to be written and the number of people to cultivate as donors. It was unanimously approved and we moved into the largest fundraising campaign of our history.

Less than three weeks later, the horror of 9-11 stopped the world.

On that morning, I was on the top floor of one of the tallest buildings in Houston, waiting for a 9 a.m. meeting with the immigration attorney. I was there to start the application process for a K-1 visa. Patrick had proposed and the next step was obtaining the visa. I, along with everyone else in the reception area, watched the television screen as the second plane hit the Twin Towers.

No one talked. No one moved. It was beyond belief.

The meeting with the attorney was a blur. He gave me papers to complete, told me the cost, explained the timeline—it would take twelve to eighteen months, but the only thing I wanted to do was get out of there and get to The Rose.

With all the death, terror, and anguish of that day, an unspeakable horror that no one could ever truly describe descended and permeated every city, every family, and every person. I remember walking around the offices, telling the employees that I loved them and asking if their families were okay. Around noon, there was a telephone call from Patrick. Nothing ever meant more to me than hearing that man's voice. I held onto the telephone receiver with both hands, assuring him I was okay, so wanting to be with him.

The September board meeting was solemn. The talk around that huge square table had little to do with The Rose or last month's meeting minutes. Listening to these thoughtful, business savvy people share their concerns, more than once hearing emotions unlike any ever shared in that room, was at times excruciating. We all hurt for our country in our own ways.

Somewhere about midway through the meeting, I brought up the capital campaign, offering to postpone it, fully expecting their agreement.

It was a total surprise when Tom said, "We should move forward. Whatever is ahead will happen. But if we stop now, I think it will take a long time to rebuild the momentum. The feasibility study was clear; we have the community's support now. No one can predict what lies ahead." As the most conservative member of the board, a banker no less, his encouragement was unexpected.

His words launched an excited and candid discussion with worst case, best case, and no case scenarios bouncing off the walls. By the end of the meeting, the motion carried to officially start the capital campaign, and we moved forward with a vengeance. That vote took courage. It was one of the most visionary decisions our board ever made, and as it turned out, one of the most painful.

For the next two months, every extra moment was consumed by the capital campaign. Maria wrote the proposals, I edited, and together we'd visit the different foundations. We were picking up steam and making some great contacts.

Then, on November 29, 2001, the headlines screamed "Enron Collapses." With $62 billion in assets, it was the largest American company ever to go bankrupt. For the next five or six months, the fallout of that collapse saturated the very fabric of our city as thousands of people lost everything, their jobs, their retirement, and their sense of hope. That loss extended into the non-profit community as folks who had benefited from Enron's generosity now scrambled to find replacement funds.

What that meant in a nutshell was another major setback to our capital campaign. Foundations wouldn't even see us at this point; they were too busy worrying over the impact on their own portfolios and the crunch of new funding requests.

In a city still crawling out from under the destruction of Tropical Storm Allison, a city where a major employer had collapsed, spawning a nosedive in the stock market, and a country that was rebounding from terrorist attacks and gearing up for war, it was insanity to be conducting a capital campaign. Our needs seemed trivial compared to all the other concerns.

We dropped our original goal from $10 million to $6 million. That step eliminated any chance of having an endowment fund for the future, but we had to give up something to make the campaign more palpable. Even $6 million wasn't enough. We wanted to pay off the building at $2.6 million, needed to purchase new equipment and furnishings at another $2 million, and most of all we had to complete the huge renovation project that encompassed over 20,000 square feet of floor space. That project could easily rack up another $2 million.

While it wasn't the first time we'd struggled to find funding, this time it was different. For every step forward, we were taking three steps backward. Each carefully written proposal, each visit with grant officers, no matter how cordial, was met with a recurring response. "Yes, we did say we would support your campaign but with the Medical Center being devastated by the storm"… or "Yes, we had pledged to provide a lead gift but the downturn of the stock market severely has impacted our portfolios."

Still, we tried. Maria assured us our Stellar Plan would inspire the wealthiest folks around to dig deep into their pockets. Yet, meeting after meeting, her reports about our progress toward actually raising money were dismal, usually falling somewhere between zero and $5,000.

Our steering committee chairperson, a dynamic and successful businessman, wasn't used to failure. During every meeting, he drilled me about our actions and couldn't understand why there was no progress. I started to dread those meetings.

The truth is that in the non-profit world, it's the board members or the campaign's steering committee who usually secure those top dollar gifts from individuals or corporations during a major fundraising campaign. At the very least, they open the doors and make the introductions. Even if our folks had been better connected with the wealthy in the community, the outcome would probably have been the same.

One large gift did come through from the Houston Endowment, and with their $500,000 we were able to make the offer on the building. We were so excited! Tom convinced the bank to loan us the rest of the money for the mortgage and extensive renovations. He secured a reasonable interest rate but it carried a balloon payment at the end of fifteen years.

After months of surveys, EPA studies, and producing financial reports, the closing day came, and on April 20, 2002, Dixie and I signed the paperwork. I left the title company with the feeling of a huge rock sitting in my stomach. We had gone from zero debt to $2.6 million. It was a big step and a scary one.

Raising money, or trying to, for the capital campaign was my primary focus. My next priority was finding another radiologist since the radiology group we were using had tired of covering our cases. "Not enough reimbursement," they said. Only slightly behind those two challenges came writing and editing grants for our daily operating needs and still running basic operations.

But in spite of all, this was a genuinely fun time. Between imagining how every nook and cranny of the building would look after the renovation and dreaming about a future with Patrick, I was truly enjoying life. Possibilities abounded!

I even toyed with the idea that once the campaign ended and the renovation project was completed, I'd go live with Patrick overseas, become an expatriate and explore the world. He reminded me then, as he has many times since, that The Rose was my first love and not one I could easily leave.

We were busy redoing the first 8,000 square foot area of the building when one of three tenants literally left in the middle of the night. Suddenly we had another 2,600 square feet of space empty, and we sure weren't prepared for that loss of rent. I countered any worries about having less money from tenant rentals with the idea that all of those areas were needed for our expansion and renovation.

Dee, my right hand person, would tease me about how excited I would get envisioning those empty spaces becoming The Rose of the future. I would come in almost every day with a new idea. I couldn't wait to gather the executive team—Dee, Amy, Pam, and Brahana— and we would launch into reworking the construction plans. Dee was my public affairs/facilities management/development director, all mixed together. She had an intriguing ability to move between appeasing and cajoling fashionable folks as they chaired events, to standing her ground with the sweatiest, grumpiest construction crew supervisor, to churning out compelling fundraising appeals with ease.

Brahana was our newcomer. She was the director of the support staff, from front desk to medical records to navigation, at both centers. Unlike Pam and Amy, who had been through many moves and remodeling projects as The Rose grew, this was the first time for Brahana. She had plenty of ideas and kept a hawk eye view on the space allotted for her folks.

"You could see it, Dorothy," Dee told me later. "I would look at the drawings, try to visualize the walls and rooms, but it seemed impossible. But you! You would talk about this area for mammography or that area for the doctors. You could see it! I watched you walk around those vacant areas. I had no idea what was going on in your mind. But you had the vision, you knew what you wanted and you made it happen."

I may have had the vision, but Dee had a lot to do with it happening. She orchestrated eighty-three different department moves and helped us get through hundreds of revisions to the plans. I had hired Dee a month before I met Patrick. A few days before she was scheduled to work, I left her a voicemail saying I was out of the country and asking if we could postpone her start date until the next week.

Dee loved to tell that story. "Out of the country?" she'd mimic. "I thought, who is this woman calling me a day before I'm supposed to start work and telling me she's leaving the country—how did that happen? What person just leaves the country? And then I found out WHY she left!" Dee would start laughing, and add, "I should have known then I was going to be working with someone who was, uh...different." Her laughter would become hysterical.

Dee was with me when I hired Blair, who warned us going in that we'd love his work but hate working with him...mainly because he was so hard to reach...which turned out to be true. He was one of five architects to bid on the renovation. His portfolio was impressive enough and, as we walked the corridors, I liked that he talked about keeping the natural light as much as possible.

Then he said, "You'll need to have a consult room off the imaging area."

I was surprised that he was a step ahead of me, and said, "How do you know that?"

He responded with, "I sat in a room just like that when my wife was diagnosed with breast cancer, she was only 29." I saw the concern that covered his face and knew he was the one who would make the dream of a first class center come true. And he did, in spite of our chronic funding dilemmas.

With all the excitement of the planning and starting to see some of the areas actually built out, the nagging reality of our finances haunted every decision. Funding had continued to dwindle, and there had not been an approval in three months. I knew every time we asked for capital campaign funds, we were sacrificing funds desperately needed for day-to-day operations.

The steering committee chairman remained unhappy and let the board know his feelings in a biting letter detailing everything I had done wrong. Thank goodness the board was supportive of me, but they also knew he had every reason to be concerned. I called him, tried to reconcile, and eventually we were able to call a truce, but on that day he wasn't talking to me about anything.

I was losing confidence that we'd raise the money to pay off the building or even have enough to finish the renovation. Each time we had to 'value engineer' some part of our construction plan and give up something I knew we'd regret later, I felt even more of a failure. We knew going in that we couldn't have everything we wanted, but so many of the nicer things, wall coverings, extra rooms to grow, specific flooring, were eliminated one by one. It was disheartening.

It was on one of those days when we had to agree to another concession, a change I had fought hard not to make, that Maria called to tell me she was leaving. Her health was failing and she had to terminate her contract. I had suspected she was ill and hated it for her. But I was equally concerned about handling the campaign without her.

During an administrative meeting later that day, I tried to maintain a 'we can do it' attitude, but no one could muster up the old enthusiasm. Returning to my office, I opened a letter from yet another funder advising that they would not be able to meet their full pledge after all: "Rebuilding the Medical Center requires our total attention and commitment, and at this time is our only priority." It was a substantial decline.

The situation, the letter, the funding decision, the call from Maria, was topped off by the radiology group telling us this was their last week to cover The Rose. It all caved in on me.

That evening I didn't share the day's events during the instant messaging e-talk with Patrick. It was too depressing to relive and go over again. Besides, what could he do about it? It didn't seem fair to him.

I did write him a note, and in it I said:

This has been another day of trying to find motivation.
It is another night of wondering what the heck I am doing, of feeling alone and wondering where I am going to get the juice to be "up"

tomorrow.

I told you that today was intense and it was. But what I couldn't tell you was that throughout all the meetings and all the events of the day, I have never felt so unsupported or undecided or weak. None of my family or friends can ever know this weakness in me and you, my Love, aren't here to tell me differently. This isn't a guilt trip. How could you ever know how stretched I have been these past years? How could I ever adequately explain how much having a home for The Rose means to me? I so wanted to secure that foundation for her, to have a place we owned to build upon, to secure The Rose's future. I love The Rose but tonight I feel like I've let her down. All my old accomplishments don't matter anymore. I don't know if I can continue to lead it.

I wondered to myself what had happened to that woman I used to be, the determined one, the one who had helped birth this place called The Rose and nurtured it along for so many years.

I went to bed, despondent and in tears. I started my nightly prayers, first asking for help for those on the prayer list, giving thanks for Patrick, the staff, friends and family.

Then I heard myself say, "Dear Lord, if you don't want me to run The Rose, then don't let me wake up in the morning."

And I meant it.

Since I woke up the next morning, I had to surmise that He or She still wanted me to run it.

So I dragged myself out of bed, dressed in my invisible suit of armor and forced smile, and journeyed off for another day of slaying dragons and looking for help under every rock and in every crevice.

In the end, the capital campaign lasted four years and raised $3.6 million. It was a glorious day in January, 2006, when we held our 'grand reopening' and toured nearly 200 folks through all the new and freshly remodeled sections. I was so proud.

In the crowd were some very special people whose personal donations pushed us forward even when the foundations were pulling back.

Months before, when Elaine and David gave me their check, she said, "We don't want The Rose to look like a clinic anymore. I don't want to see chairs lined up and down the hallway! I want you to use this money on your reception area. Make it look nice." And it did. For the first time in our history the furniture all matched. From the granite on the counters to dark wood paneling to the copper accents throughout the room, everything looked classy. The room was large, spacious, and ready for even the most discerning patient. Elaine was a survivor and patient of Dixie's, and that event marked the beginning of many years of their support. Elaine still comes to The Rose once a year and brings a check with her.

The gift from Donita and Jim was also major. Donita wanted to buy one of our mammography machines because, as she explained, "If it never breaks, then I'll never break."

My heart sank because I knew that the cancer Donita was fighting was one of the really bad ones. I countered with, "Donita, you can't afford one of our machines, but why don't you let us use your gift for a special room, a family meeting or consult room?" She loved that idea and absolutely glowed when I walked her and Jim into the room. Its soft green walls, shiny wooden sofa table and nice chairs were inviting. A beautiful quilt, made by a local Girl Scout troop in honor of The Rose and our survivors, hung on the wall and gave the room a cozy feeling.

I visited Donita at her home a week before she died. She was in bed with blankets piled high over her and the paraphernalia of illness cluttered every flat surface in the room. I rubbed her feet, doubled socked because she was so cold. Even then, she talked about how her newest treatment was bound to work. Even then, she didn't want to break.

So our campaign ended. While we had our own building, it still had a mortgage on it and unfortunately we didn't have one penny set aside to maintain it and nothing to fall back on.

The night when I had prayed to not wake up, I already knew in my heart that the capital campaign would turn out to be both a success and a failure. If the campaign had been successful, it could have marked a time of moving toward financial solvency. Instead, by not reaching even our minimum goal, we would face the years ahead always being one step behind and always struggling against having a year-end deficit.

I still remember the sound of Patrick's voice when we had our weekly talk over the phone and the way he gasped when I finally told him the story of that day and about my prayer.

"You prayed to not wake up? What on earth were you thinking? Are you crazy?" he asked, his tone incredulous.

That night, I probably was.

Chapter 17
Doctors Come in All Sizes

The woman sitting across the table from me was someone I knew well. Carol had been our physicist for years, completing the annual inspection of our many pieces of equipment. Her review was among the many requirements of law. The MQSA law, backed by the FDA, could carry stiff fines, up to and including closure, if her first sweep of our equipment was not up to standards.

Every physicist review was critical and Carol was the most critical of all reviewers. She dressed simply and for comfort, her style, like her mannerisms, was reserved, never flashy. But the sharpness in her eyes and the range of her vocabulary gave away the fact that she was indeed a highly trained, incredibly intelligent scientist.

"Believe me, if it wasn't for the work you do, I would never come out here on evenings or weekends!"

I nodded, remembering that she and the team had worked last Friday and Saturday and it was Easter weekend.

She continued, "I knew I had to get those surveys done! I'd never do that for the for-profits, but I sure didn't want The Rose to be closed."

"Gosh, Carol, we really do appreciate it; you've always understood how important it is to us to not lose a single day."

"The Rose is very dear to me." Tears welled up in her eyes and she reached for a tissue, "You may not remember this, but my mother died of breast cancer when I was fifteen. There was nothing they could do." She stopped, blew her nose, and stayed lost in those sad memories for a few minutes. I reached out and touched her arm.

"That is one reason why it is so important to me that The Rose be the best it can be. You do breast cancer the right way, it's about the patients, not the money!" Her tone was abrupt, serious. "I cover all the major medical centers and everywhere I go someone tells me a story about sending a woman to you...believe me, every technologist in this town knows how good you are. They know they can call you for that uninsured woman. Do you realize that?"

Before I could respond, she said, "And do you also realize that you have one of the most renowned radiologists in the nation in Ward Parsons?" She smiled. "Do you have any idea how many of the radiologists in Houston have attended one of his seminars? They all speak so highly of him."

After struggling through years of the revolving door of radiologists and all their different eccentricities, we had almost given up hope of finding the right one. So it was with a healthy dose of cynicism that I approached the first interview with Ward Parsons in May of 2003. Amy, on the other hand, was absolutely ecstatic.

Ward loves to tell the story of how Amy persuaded him to come to The Rose.

"Amy is too short a name for someone so accomplished," he laughed. "She should be Amy the Magnificent. I encountered Amy many times over the years at various conferences. At every meeting she would ask, 'When are you coming to be our radiologist?'

"She included me as a guest speaker at several of The Rose's seminars for mammography technologists. Every time I spoke, she asked the question. After one seminar, she gave me a small stuffed teddy bear wearing a Western hat and a black necktie labeled "Houston." She added a pink ribbon pin as a tie tack. And of course she asked, 'When are you coming to be our radiologist?'

"After several years in Dallas, I decided on a career change. I interviewed in many places, but none seemed quite right. Then I remembered Amy. How could I forget? I called her and asked, 'Are you still looking for a radiologist for The Rose.' Her immediate answer was, 'Yes, when can you start?' That concluded the longest and shortest interview I ever had," he smiled.

Ward is a curious soul. His journey to becoming a doctor started with him being an ultrasound technologist, and he always insisted on doing his own scanning long after he became the world famous radiologist. His professional career was launched while serving in the Navy, and his transition from military to academic life landed him a position as one of the top professors at Southwestern University. Ward taught the radiology residents and trained many future radiologists.

Even though I had seen pictures of Ward lecturing at the seminars, I was not prepared for this giant of a man when I first met him in my office. He easily stood six foot four inches tall, with a massive body to match. When he came through the door, his bulk literally filled up the entire opening. The moment he entered, the room suddenly felt smaller. His long torso made him almost as tall sitting down as some people are standing up. Looking at him sitting in one of my small chairs, at least for his frame, there was only one thought that ran through my mind, *How in the world will this man fit into all our tiny exam rooms?*

We exchanged pleasantries, and out of nowhere he said, "I know what you must be thinking."

"You do?" I said, caught completely off-guard.

"You're wondering if I'll intimidate the women. I know I'm a big person," he smiled, easy with his words. "I learned a long time ago that when I go into an exam room, I have to sit down. That way I'm at the same level as the woman who is on the exam table, we are eye to eye when I'm talking to her. I make sure of that. The last thing a woman needs when she is having an ultrasound or biopsy is to have some big guy like me towering over her. She's already frightened enough."

I liked his approach, but the words that stood out most to me from that interview were the "when I'm talking to her."

None of the other radiologists were crazy about talking to patients, at least not in the early 2000s. The last radiologist, who had left us high and dry, daily whined that "these women act like I'm their personal doctor!" He huffed that he couldn't possibly "take on that kind of liability." He complained when they asked medical questions, saying that he "wasn't about to be put in that position, especially by an uninsured woman."

I wanted to scream at him, "Hell yes they act like you're their doctor. Most of those women haven't had the luxury of seeing a real doctor in four or five years!"

But Ward didn't talk that way and, true to his character, he didn't act that way either. He saw more than a patient on the exam table, he saw a woman who was scared and concerned. It didn't matter if she was rich or poor or in-between.

Most folks had no idea how difficult it was to recruit radiologists who were dedicated to breast imaging. Of the 20,000 physicians who graduated every year, only 2,000 would go into breast imaging, and even those would insist they needed to be doing other interventional diagnostic radiology to ensure their financial security. An MRI netted $300 or $400 a pop, a mammogram maybe $40. It was all about reimbursement and the number of procedures they would have to do to make the money they wanted to make.

Even though they were hard to find, I grew weary listening to the docs who earned four to five hundred thousand dollars a year from mammography whine about how they barely made enough to ensure a good life for their family or pay for their malpractice insurance. They had no overhead costs working for The Rose, so try as I might to understand their plight, it didn't compute.

Besides no overhead and being well paid, every physician who ever contracted with us had other streams of income. Dixie had income from her private practice and surgery, one short-lived radiologist had his own tele-radiography business, and Ward was a well-paid key lecturer at physician seminars. Believe me, I didn't care how much they made, but whenever we had a slow month, they were the first ones in my office wanting to know what I was going to do about it. Every sponsored woman's procedures included paying the physician's interpretation fees, so finding funding or driving insured women into the centers fell to me and my team. In the end, it is always about the money, just like every other working stiff in this world.

I have to admit, the changes Ward made in our processes brought The Rose to a higher level of care and made him worth every penny. He was a specialist in mammography, he wasn't some guy who read ten or fifteen mammograms part of the day and then went off to do upper GIs or look at chest x-rays. His recall rate was among the lowest in the nation, wavering around 5%. He knew what he was looking at and he took a stand—either it was normal or abnormal—telling the woman to return for her annual in twelve months or that she needed an immediate work-up. Six month follow-ups were almost non-existent in his recommendations. His low recall rate was great for the women and our reputation—the last radiologist had hovered around a 17-19% recall rate, which didn't sit well with our referring physicians.

He initiated "same day diagnosis," an unheard of approach. Back then, the standard process could involve a fifteen or seventeen day wait by the time the radiologist read the images, the report was dictated and transcribed, then mailed to the referring physician, who eventually reviewed the recommendation and called the patient with her results.

When a woman had a diagnostic exam, she knew something was going on in her body that could turn out to be cancer. The anxiety of waiting created major stress. That was a stress Ward eliminated during the first month he was with us. When he completed the exam, he showed the films to each patient and explained what was going on. If it was a cyst, he could aspirate it or it would simply go away on its own. If it was something suspicious, then a biopsy was scheduled.

He was right. Women can handle most anything; just don't make them wait forever for a report. The patients loved his approach, loved the time he took explaining the nuances of their breast tissue, loved the way he genuinely cared.

But one of the most courageous steps he took was going to bat for Dixie so she could officially read mammograms and be reimbursed for it. At that time, Dixie came to The Rose a couple of days a week to do ultrasounds or biopsies on her patients. But the days of her performing those long surgeries and standing for hours over an operating table had taken a toll on her back. Dixie often talked about 'someday' when she would be able to work at The Rose full time.

Besides, she pointed out, she could give The Rose that extra help we needed and make a whole lot more money reading mammograms. She was right. As unfair as it seems, a radiologist reading films made more than she did cutting someone's body open and doing a lumpectomy. Declining reimbursement continues to snap at the heels of physicians and it's no wonder so many are leaving the profession.

But working with us full time meant that she had to be certified to read mammograms.

It didn't take much talking for me to show Ward that we needed extra help, at the rate we were growing he would never catch up. But even after he agreed to the idea of having another person around to help read, it took a little longer to convince him that help could be Dixie.

A surgeon reading mammograms was unusual, but Dixie wouldn't be the first one certified to do it. Still, the imaging world belonged to the radiologists and they balked at any other type of doctor reading films. The orthopods had gotten around it, as had some chiropractors, but surgeons? That idea really made the fur fly. The only way a surgeon was allowed to read mammograms was if he or she worked under the supervision of a radiologist.

Few radiologists then, or now, are comfortable with that solution. But Ward did what was best for The Rose.

He signed off on Dixie's first 250 official mammograms, she took some additional courses in radiation safety, and Amy made sure all the paperwork was done correctly. Soon Dixie was on our license. Ward took a lot of flak from his colleagues because of her reading. One even sent a letter of complaint to leaders in the radiology arena and always made a point in his ads that only radiologists were reading films at his place.

But none of that mattered to our referring doctors. They were confident in Dixie's skills and patients loved being seen by her.

Soon our volume exceeded what Ward and Dixie could manage and we had to recruit other radiologists—sometimes we were lucky to find the ones like Ward, who weren't afraid to be a doctor to our patients.

It was during this time that another doctor came into our lives: Dr. Peggy Connor. She wasn't there to read mammograms, but she was there to make a difference.

Peggy had just returned from Mexico to care for her ailing

mother. With four years of medical training at Guadalajara Medical School behind her, she needed to complete another year doing community work. It was her final requirement to becoming a physician in Mexico. She applied for our sponsorship coordinator job and Brahana was determined that we hire her. I had strong reservations about a doctor, even one who wasn't licensed in the States, ever being happy doing a clerical job. Boy, was I wrong!

Peggy, like Ward, had a presence that was all her own. Imagine the solid body of a football linebacker, mixed with the deftness of a Native American Indian warrior, contained within a black lace-covered and tiara'ed Senorita hiding her face demurely behind an open fan. Peggy had these shoulders, too broad for her short frame, that sat squarely atop a nicely proportioned, full busted and full hipped figure. Her penetrating clear blue eyes, framed by thick sharply arched eyebrows, gleamed with the fierceness of a hunter about to pounce upon its prey. Her shiny long blond hair, piled high on her head, made her look regal with a touch of old time Hollywood glamor. Her face had a defined square shape to it, her jaw was strong and jutted out, her creamy complexion was flawless, and when she smiled, which was often, she was beautiful.

If her appearance was confusing, the way she processed information was equally off-putting. One never knew where Peggy was coming from or where she was going once she got there, yet more often than not, she made sense…eventually.

There was no question she was intelligent. She could never have finished medical school in another country, handling assignments and tests in a foreign language, or graduated from Texas A & M with honors without brains.

Peggy never returned to Mexico after her mother died. She bought a farm in Central Texas and was happy being one with nature. But when we needed someone to perform breast examinations for our uninsured women going through the Breast and Cervical Cancer Services state program, she returned. One week of each month, she worked at The Rose and had a chance to use all those years of medical training.

Sometimes Peggy acted like a doctor, sometimes she didn't. But for those uninsured patients she examined and guided into service, she was always the physician in charge. When she spoke to them, they listened; they trusted her and were remarkably compliant in showing up for tests. And they told her their stories.

It was Peggy who noticed the international quality among our sponsored patients. For weeks she meticulously tracked every patient's birth home and presented the list to me. They came from Columbia,

Cuba, Ecuador, Egypt, El Salvador, Guatemala, Honduras, Mexico, Nigeria, Vietnam, Pakistan, India, Iran, and Iraq, as well as Ohio, Arkansas, Maine, and Missouri in the United States. Truly, need isn't isolated to any single country and encompasses all cultures. And, more often than not, when we diagnosed an undocumented woman, she wasn't from Mexico.

Peggy would end her week at The Rose by sending me stories of her patients via inter-office email. Some were unbelievably sad; others were brimming with inspiration. It was those stories that kept me connected to our patients and often kept me awake at night. Many tugged at my heart but one will stay in my treasure trove of special notes forever.

> *Dorothy,*
>
> *It's another Blessed week and I find myself once again at the Galleria location listening to incredible stories. This one I could not pass up, please add it to your file of "reality" and pull from it if it ever is of use. If we could somehow get a grant for International Women's Affairs, our women would "win" with their stories.*
>
> *In the patient interview of medical history, Maria stated that she was from Nuevo Laredo, Mexico, and reported she had a personal history of cervical cancer that was treated with a hysterectomy. She told me the following story:*
>
> *"My mother committed suicide when I was fourteen ... there were five children ... my father left us to start a new life and I was on my own. I lived by myself and tried to find work. When I went about asking for work, two "family friends" (different men on two different occasions) offered to put me up in an apartment as their amante (lover). I did not want to be a kept woman so I lived in poverty ... scratching to make a living. I met a man, tried to have a life, but after a while he left. By 1992, I had three children, one was nine, one seven, and one was two weeks old.*
>
> *I had lived in that border town until I turned 25 when I decided to SWIM ACROSS THE RIVER. I had a sister who lived in Houston. So ... because I was a really good swimmer, one night I held on to the two older children, put the two week old child on a raft, and swam across the Rio Grande River. I had nothing but the clothes on my back and my children. Different people on the US side of the border took me in and got me to Houston. I didn't know them."*
>
> *Roll the tape forward, 22 years later, to 2014 ... her three children are doing well; working and raising families and paying taxes, they have each made a life for themselves, all naturalized citizens. While they care for their mother, she continues to work at odd jobs "sending her father who is in poor health" money whenever she can ... so that HE can eat.*

This woman is AMAZING! We have the most incredible "roll call" of heroes in our ranks.
I love my job!
Dr. Peggy

Chapter 18
Gift Giving

I knew something was wrong the moment I entered the ultrasound room. Dixie was sitting in her usual place on the tall stool next to the very end of the counter, her back touching the wall, pen poised over paperwork. A patient's chart lay open in front of her; films were neatly stacked on one side, colored sheets of paper on the other. A few feet away, the tech bustled around the end of the exam table, quietly stripping off the protective covering. She then turned to the metal movable stand where a biopsy tray, its tools spent and disposables used, sat waiting to be cleaned and restocked.

Dixie sat motionless. Her eyes were dull. She stared at nothing, her gaze reaching out beyond the paperwork. The pen in her hand continued to hover.

"Dixie?" I said. No answer. I glanced at the tech; she shook her head and shrugged her shoulders.

"Dixie?" I stepped closer to her and noticed the dark circles under her eyes. It had been a long week, a long day. We scheduled most of our ultrasound-guided biopsies on Fridays; it was the only day of the week when we could count on Dixie being there for the entire day. On this Friday, fifteen women were scheduled, nine of them did not have insurance.

I moved directly in front of her. Startled, she looked up and at that moment huge tears filled her eyes.

"What's wrong, Dixie?"

She shook her head and looked down. "Did you see that young Spanish girl? The one we just did the biopsy on? She's 24. She has two children. There's no doubt," Dixie nodded toward the exam table, "it's definitely cancer and it's bad. Another young girl that we are sending to the UTMB. Did you see the look in her eyes? She's so frightened. She's terrified." Her words trailed off.

Silence punched through the room. I waited.

"I tried to reassure her," she began again, more to herself than to me, "I told her everything would be all right. But I know what is about to happen to her. She'll be just another procedure—another troll; another test subject for the interns. There is no telling what will happen to her, to her body, after they get through practicing on her. She'll never look right again. She'll never get over it. I remember how horrified the women were when they saw their bodies for the first time, how ugly the surgeries were."

Dixie stopped. Her eyes darted around the room. A look of relief crossed her face. I wasn't sure if the look was because she was glad the tech had left the room or glad she hadn't been whisked back in time, reliving her days as a surgical intern.

"I know, I know," she went on, waving her hand toward the door. "I should be glad she's getting treatment." She wiped her eyes with the back of her hand. "I just remember how that felt, how it felt to be treated like a nobody, like a troll. I remember being on that gurney, big as a blimp, lying there in the hallway with all these people going back and forth, talking about me like I wasn't there. *The ignorant one that hadn't had any prenatal care, the uninsured one, the stupid one.* They let me lie there the entire night. I was so alone. I'd never had a baby before."

I had heard this story before, of Dixie being dropped off by her husband at the charity hospital and finding her way to the emergency room to have her first child, a son who didn't arrive until eighteen hours later.

"I know how that young woman is going to feel; alone, like a nobody," Dixie sighed, her lips formed a tight line. "At least I could speak English," she whispered.

Silence hung between us. The scenes of the day, the whole week, rolled together and ended in the one that had just played out in this eight by ten foot room.

A young woman with few options. A young woman facing cancer. A young woman who had kids at home, who couldn't possibly grasp the journey ahead. Even if she could understand the language, the technical jargon would go over her head, as it did most everyone. No one would be there to hold her hand as she went into surgery, no one would be very worried about her emotional health.

Nothing could prepare her for the transition from the woman she was today to the one she would become or be reduced to in a matter of only a few weeks.

I reached for Dixie's hand and squeezed it. For moments, we were lost in that young woman's future. A tapping at the door forced us to the present, to the work at hand.

"Someday, Dorothy," Dixie straightened her back and pulled

herself up, standing to greet the next patient. "Someday, we're going to have our own hospital. We'll take care of women like her. And we'll do it the right way."

We hugged.

"Yes, Dixie," I promised. "Someday."

That promise is one that I have not been able to keep.

There were plenty of hospitals around; there wasn't a need for another one and they were all vying for the same meager insured dollar. If anything, we needed a Rose in every hospital, vying for the dignity of patients, which in my book meant not having to grovel for healthcare at the very time they were both physically and mentally most vulnerable.

We needed a place where even poor people were treated like human beings. I will never understand why poverty has become such a stigma in our country. Ironically, it is no longer about the haves and have nots; now there is a huge population of 'used to haves' that 'don't have anymore.'

From what I've seen, there is no greater prejudice than the attitudes displayed to poor people—race or gender or age no longer separate us the way wealth does.

Every sponsored woman we serve has been pushed into unimaginably difficult situations, coping with few resources and fewer places to turn for help. In the end, they are left woefully unequipped and mentally and physically exhausted. By the time they come to The Rose, the boulders of responsibilities in their knapsack of life have become too heavy to carry. We can't move all the rocks out of their way, but by God, we can help with at least one of those boulders.

For many of our sponsored women, English is not their first language. While they can communicate, the nuances of different cultures add another stone to that knapsack.

Regardless of one's first language, when the diagnosis of cancer is made, every person is thrown into the foreign land of the medical world, with words and phrases as alien as any exotic language.

Most of our women are the primary wage earners, heads of household and responsible for dependent children—most often alone. I am outrageously annoyed by the term 'single mother,' they sure didn't get pregnant by themselves, but most of the time it is the mother who finds herself caring for the kids alone. Coping with language barriers, not having consistent medical care, being the single head of a household, those factors were common denominators, at least they were until around 2008 when the economy went south. That's when the most common denominator among the people turning to The Rose for help became that they had had jobs within the past two years (with insurance), and then they didn't.

I don't need the stories of our sponsored women to know what being poor looks like. I only need to think of my sister and look back on all the years she has struggled. Mavis had four kids before age 25. When she made the break from her husband, she was left to care for those same kids, and with no education or other support, she managed. Even then, she wasn't healthy, and having no insurance kept her that way.

Poor is working fifty hours a week at Whataburger, but still not having enough take home pay because the only way the kids could eat that week was by charging meals against your account.

Poor is not being able to accept a quarter an hour pay raise because it would mean your juvenile diabetic child would no longer qualify for Medicaid.

Poor means being in the emergency room about once a month for a chronic disease because you can't afford the medicine the doctor ordered for you the last time you were admitted.

Poor is wishing you could smile but the years of neglect have rotted out your front teeth and turned them into dark ragged caves of cavities.

Poor is staying in hell because there is no other choice.

Poor is watching your children live in that same hell.

Poor is wondering how to pay for the funeral of a 22-year-old daughter who was killed in a tragic car accident early one Monday morning. My sister's only daughter, the light of her life, miscalculated a curve on an icy road on her way to work. She left behind a two-year-old and now my sister manages his care on social security benefits of $800 a month.

My sister never had to fight breast cancer, yet her disease was just as life threatening, made all the more terminal by poverty.

Hers is the kind of poor no amount of family help can solve, especially when a health issue erupts, then the system sucks the very life out of a soul. If the systems and the bureaucracy don't totally succeed, then the worry is sure to. Worry was her constant companion.

For some of the women we've served, the most difficult care to get is hospice. Once treatment no longer works and the cancer has 'won,' Medicaid coverage stops—no more medical treatment equals no longer having the ability to qualify for Medicaid.

Without Medicaid, there isn't any coverage for hospice; without hospice, people die at home (if they still have a home at this point) or in a friend or loved one's home. Few end in charity hospitals, those beds are needed for the living. How sad that even the ability to die in dignity is stolen. Even finding the slightest relief from pain depends on an insurance status.

Why would anyone ever believe a person would 'choose' this way of living or dying?

The women I know still love and care and hug and find reasons to hope, they love being with their families, enjoy an occasion to dress up or a chance to visit with a friend. I marvel watching my sister laugh at her grandchild's antics, share her pride in dressing him for his first day of school, and I cry every time she says "half my heart is in heaven." She's my hero.

Like all the sponsored women we serve, that ability to continue in spite of…finish the sentence, the list is long…defies all logic. Theirs is a courage I can't quite fathom, never could grasp, and always admired. They find a way to get through, somehow.

I had witnessed that courage often, but there was one time in December, 2009, when it took on a deeper meaning. The Holidays were pretty tough for our women, most worked, juggled home and children, and were fighting the physical effects of the treatment, which can be pretty difficult. Money was never in surplus, and when work hours and pay got cut because of time off needed for chemotherapy, Holiday presents for the little ones were out of reach.

For many years, our patient navigators organized a Holiday party for the children of our women who had been diagnosed during the previous year. It was an annual tradition and our employees gathered gift ideas, clothes sizes, and items needed from the families and found people to be 'angels' to fill those wants and needs.

Corkey, one of our board members, brought a crew from his Casa Ole restaurant and all the fixings for a great Mexican lunch. Holiday decorations brightened the tables; over a hundred chairs lined the walls, transforming our lobby into a huge fiesta.

Those parties were joyful times, watching the kids' eyes light up when a bike or an iPod or a complete doll set were brought out, hearing the gleeful shouts, and seeing the shy ones' precious smiles as they accepted a bright and shiny package.

Mothers would try to hide the tears slipping down their cheeks. They too received gifts, but I knew the tears were for the children. This was a special occasion and everyone dressed up. Kids dashed around wearing freshly pressed Sunday best clothes. Most of the women wore scarfs or wigs to hide bald heads.

But during that party, I saw more than the normal amount of dark circles under eyes and drawn faces behind those smiles. Worry was in the air. People were still scraping out from under September's Hurricane Ike, a disaster that devastated the city. The banking crisis had hit and folks in general brooded over the economy doing its nosedive. While the media ceaselessly harped on an uncertain future, these women faced the New Year wondering if they would see another Christmas, a child graduate, a new grandchild.

I moved through the crowd when Nyla, our data analysis manager, stopped me. She introduced me to a woman from Pakistan, Ms. Pano, who was wearing the traditional clothing of her country, her sari and scarf ample cover for a body forever changed and not yet recovered from surgery.

I asked the usual questions: "Where are you in your recovery?" "How are you feeling?" but this lady had something important, according to Nyla, to say to me. As Nyla continued to translate from Urdu, I started feeling uncomfortable, almost embarrassed. This woman's words of praise were so genuine, her thankfulness palpable.

"The Rose saved my life," she said, taking my hand and pulling it to her face. She kissed it before I could stop her. "I felt so alone, there was no one to help me, I was so afraid. Thank you for starting this wonderful place."

Her story unfolded. As she told it in her language, Nyla translated. In December, 2008, she and her husband and four sons were preparing to come to The United States for the first time on an immigrant visa. But along with the excitement of relocation, she had found a lump in her breast. With no family history, she ignored it, thinking it was due to stress and all the hard work of the move. When they arrived in the US, their struggles began. When she told her relatives about the lump, she was told that she would not be able to get any kind of healthcare.

"I still remember touching the lump with my hand, feeling helpless and scared. I was scared about my family and I was scared about my life. Day by day, I could feel it grow bigger and my fears grew with it. I was sure that this lump would lead to death. I did not know where to turn," Nyla continued, translating Ms. Pano's story.

"When my oldest son found work, he met a young doctor who volunteered at a local clinic. My son told him about my situation and he told my son to rush me to Al Shifa Clinic, where Dr. Haq saw patients on Sundays.

"Dr. Haq sent me to The Rose. They took real good care of me. Before my mammogram, when they saw me wearing my abaya over my dress, they gave me a long gown that would touch my feet. When the cancer was diagnosed, they found me treatment.

"It has been a year since I found the lump. I had surgery, then chemotherapy, and now radiation." Nyla's voice was husky as she translated Ms. Pano's last words, "Even though they do not speak my language at The Rose, they speak the universal language of care and the language of love for humanity."

I marveled at the chance meeting of her son and the doctor. Angels truly were at work in her story.

During that same Holiday party there was one woman who sat off by herself, she stared out over the crowd, her eyes unfocused. She held her little bag of goodies tightly, and from the way her head jerked up when I approached, it was obvious I had startled her. I sat beside her and learned that her daughter-in-law had died recently in a tragic car wreck. She was trying to care for her three grandchildren while recovering from her own surgery.

"This will not be a very happy Christmas for those young'uns. We just don't have any extra money," she said.

"I so wish we had known," I responded, saying we could have added them to our list. She assured me that The Rose finding her treatment was more than enough and patted her bag of goodies while thanking me for inviting her to the party.

The next morning, for some unknown reason, I looked out my window. From the second floor, I watched as a scene unfolded below me. A man was unloading boxes filled with wrapped presents and two new bikes, moving them from the back of one pickup truck to another.

It was Corkey! *That's odd*, I thought.

Then I saw our patient, the grandmother I had visited with the day before. She exited her truck, walked hurriedly around its side, and gave him a big hug. Her smile was huge and I could almost hear her thanks through the closed windows.

Later we learned that he had overheard her conversation and taken her aside, asking if she could meet him the next morning. That's so like Corkey. Except for my chance spotting of him, we never would have known the story of him being Santa to those kids.

Yes, The Rose offers vital medical services: biopsies, access to treatment, support groups. All are very important in the never-ending fight against breast cancer.

But the help of one human being to another over a rough patch in life can be as rich with hope as any treatment.

Chapter 19
A Rose is Not Always The Rose

Having a name like The Rose has not always been easy.

In fact, having the word rose in our name has created a lot of confusion. One time I checked the yellow pages and found over 24 companies with the word rose in their name. We were confused with everything from The Rose Florist to the Rose on Richmond, a rowdy popular bar in the trendiest part of Houston in the late '90s. That was when Constable Bill Bailey showed up at Dixie's office with a subpoena for back property taxes, ready to arrest her. Dixie called me saying I needed to hightail it over to her place pronto to explain to him our organization didn't pay taxes...not like those.

If being confused with flower shops and bars wasn't bad enough, when our name was associated with other non-profits it brought PR nightmares. That fact became obvious when I was at an event for a pretty elite business women's network. It was all social, with women welcoming newbies like me, catching up with old colleagues and enjoying the evening of wine and cheese.

I'm never any good at small talk but was doing my best to mingle. I was delighted by the number of women who knew about The Rose and I fussed over those who told me that they came to us for their mammograms. But there were more women who didn't know us, and as the night wore on, I had to explain one too many times that The Rose wasn't one of the other non-profits that had the word rose in its name.

"Oh, The Rose. That's the foundation for the physician who died!" one woman exclaimed. "I supported the Run for The Roses!" Seeing the look on my face, she added, "Isn't that yours?"

"That's a wonderful organization," I responded, and meant it. "It was started to honor Dr. Marnie Rose and to raise money for brain cancer. We are a breast cancer organization."

Another one said, "Oh, I know Cindy and all the great work she does since her sister's diagnosis. I understand Franklin donates a lot of surgeries to your poor women. He is such a wonderful plastic surgeon." She was talking about the Rose Ribbon Foundation.

"Yes, he did do one surgery that I am aware of," I said with a smile.

There was someone who confused us with Steven Rose, a radiologist who specialized in mammography. I acknowledged that we certainly knew him, in fact he'd worked for us at one time—"only part time," I added. It was ironic, there had been so much confusion with us, probably due to all the great publicity we had had lately. Our name had become a problem for him, and his group had recently changed their name.

But one response stopped me cold. A woman joined the group I was standing in; someone introduced me, noting that I was 'with' The Rose.

She exclaimed, "The Rose? Oh, I know all about The Rose and how Jim Rose got it started."

"Jim Rose?" I asked, totally taken off-guard. I'd fielded comments about the other organizations many times in the past, but this was a first.

"Jim Rose started the Rose?" I repeated, incredulous. Jim was Dixie's ex-husband.

She nodded, "I know him very well. I know all about how he provided the seed money to get The Rose off the ground. I've been friends with him and his wife, Pam, for years."

I could have let it go. I could have said something polite or been more generous, but this was one time I couldn't. Something valuable was at stake, a piece of our history I simply could not deny.

What got The Rose off the ground sure wasn't Jim Rose's money, but an award that brought Dixie and our dream the kind of publicity most folks can barely imagine and we could never have afforded.

It was the summer of 1985 when I nominated Dixie for the Women on the Move award, a contest created by the Texas Executive Women and the *Houston Post* to recognize ten outstanding women in the community. Since I was Dixie's number one fan, filling up the three pages of narrative describing the candidate and explaining why she should receive the award was easy.

Dixie's personal story had already hit the local newspaper, but I never imagined the impact it would have once it appeared in the number one newspaper of the fourth largest city in the US. It wasn't the kind of story heard every day; it certainly didn't have the normal background connected to the journey of becoming a medical doctor.

True, in the mid-'80s, being the second female surgeon to finish the surgical residency program at UTMB-Galveston at a time when less than 3% of all physicians were women was newsworthy. But her real media appeal was the way she championed a little known disease like breast cancer. She publicly promoted screening and early detection, while her doctor colleagues challenged her, "What is all the fuss about? We only see two or three breast cancer cases a year."

"Forget the mammogram," was their primary argument, "it's costly and unproven. Just wait until you can feel the lump and then take it out."

Dixie would really go ballistic hearing that rationale.

It was my job to feed the press news releases, and the opening of Bayshore Hospital's breast imaging center was no exception. Of course, I centered the story around Dr. Dixie Mclillo, expert on breast cancer.

Dixie's personal story didn't become common knowledge until an interview with Clara Clay, reporter for the *Pasadena Citizen*. Clara had spent an hour with Dixie, meticulously recording facts and figures about breast cancer incidence and mortality, listening to Dixie recite the steps of breast self-exam and nuances of mammograms.

Clara turned off the recorder and posited a simple question. "You are so passionate about this, Dr. Dixie. What made you want to be a doctor?" she asked.

Dixie, thinking everything was now 'off the record,' started talking, and Clara spent another hour with her, never taking a note.

The next day, the headline of the *Pasadena Citizen* read "Local Surgeon Overcomes Rough Beginnings as a High School Drop-Out." The article detailed every word Dixie had shared with Clara.

There it was in black and white. The story recounted Dixie being 'kicked out' of high school at age sixteen and how she went on to marry young and have another child by the time she was eighteen years old. Realizing she couldn't even get a job at the five and dime without a diploma, she returned to Amarillo Caprock High School and finished. With her mother watching the kids, she went on to community college.

The best part of her story about getting into medical school was the gift of her OB/GYN, Dr. Wyatt. Learning that her grade point average was 3.9, he nixed her dreams of being a lab technician and encouraged her to take the MCAT and apply for medical school. He even paid for the test so she wouldn't have any excuses not to try. Sure enough, her scores were competitive, but being accepted into any of the state supported medical colleges was going to be a long shot.

Dixie's interviews for medical school were another story. The first interviewer told her, "Someone ought to kick your butt. The idea that you'd even apply for medical school and take up the place that ought to go to a man. The only thing you want to do is find some rich doctor and get married, and then all the money the state spends on you will be wasted, down the tubes." He dismissed her, as did her second interviewer at another college.

By interview number three, Dixie had had enough. She walked into that doctor's office saying, "I want you to understand one thing: I will be a doctor! I don't want to hear about my needing to stay home with my children. I went to high school with these boys, and to college with these boys, and I can damn sure go to medical school with these boys. Now, if you don't accept me I'll go back and get my Masters and reapply, and if you still won't accept me, I'll get my PhD and I'll come back, but I guarantee you I will get into medical school!"

Dr. Lorrentz, the interviewer, threw his hand up in front of his face and said, "Slow down, Lady, I didn't even say hello."

The story of Dixie's entry into the medical world was included in my nomination for the TEW award. She was selected from over 400 other nominations as one of the top ten Women on the Move.

No other single event impacted The Rose's beginning more than that. Full-page feature articles, all in color, appeared in the Houston newspaper. People clamored to have her as keynote speaker and she made the rounds as guest physician for the radio shows and local TV spots. She never looked better or was more compelling. Becoming a blond suited her and she wore a lot of red. The award gave her a very visible public platform to talk about this dream we shared, a dream called The Rose, a place where no one was turned away, where a woman could receive screening regardless of her ability to pay.

As sometimes happens to successful women, this award had a down side. It seemed the more of a 'public' figure Dixie became, the farther apart she and Jim grew. He didn't come to the Women on the Move awards luncheon. But as life seems to work for Dixie, she stayed friends with him. Even as an ex-husband, Jim brought in one of the higher bids when he was 'sold' during our first fundraiser, the Bachelors of Distinction Auction.

So I turned to the woman who was so adamant about knowing The Rose's beginning, and said, "I remember now, Jim was one of the bachelors at our first fundraiser. He didn't have much else to do with our beginning." She frowned, but I continued before she could speak. "Believe me, I'm a co-founder. Dr. Melillo and I started The Rose in 1986 with a handful of volunteers and a little money from that fundraiser...very little...only $7,000." I stressed the 'little' and genuinely laughed, "We rounded up every bachelor we knew, doctors, lawyers, and bankers to auction them off. It was our start."

I shared more stories about that night, and soon she and the other women were absorbed in the tales and all were laughing.

These days when I say, "I'm with The Rose," most folks know which organization I mean. Some tell me we helped a friend or loved one. Occasionally, someone will say, "I know The Rose well. You saved my life."

Chapter 20
Too Pretty

Tommye's hands shook as she handed me the sheets of paper and an envelope. She was our assistant accountant and handled the daily mail. Her words were halting, coming from someplace deep inside. "This one," she said, "will make you cry." She shrugged, "At least it did me. I can't imagine a husband would care so much…" her words trailed and she turned her head away, but not soon enough. I saw the gleam of tears in her eyes.

I turned to the papers and started reading: "This donation is being made by my company in honor of my wife. She is now a seven-year survivor." The words continued, documenting her struggles and triumphs and how much they appreciated The Rose. There was a photograph of a happy, middle-aged woman wearing a tee-shirt, looking directly into the camera. Traces of the chemo treatment were obvious, the cap of an eighth of an inch of hair growing back, the slight puffiness, but most of all was that unmistakable glow of a women who believes she's never going to have to sit through another IV drip again.

The donation was a nice one. To The Rose, all donations are nice, but this one was really nice and I silently thanked the Universe that brought this to us—to me—on this day. God has a way of reminding me—at the very moment I get too involved in the 'business' end of our work—what the real business of The Rose is all about.

I smiled thinking about all the letters that I had saved over the years. My personal little treasure trove filled up a couple of drawers in the credenza. I knew I would scan this one and share it with the staff, but before I did that, before I made the call to the husband, before I wrote the thank you note, I granted myself a few moments of reflection.

Letters like this one, from women or families or friends, feel like invisible hands gently reaching out to us and, with a firm shake of the shoulders, announcing, "Pay Attention! Here it is! This is why! Don't forget!"

On this day, I moved back in time. We had never had many responses from our uninsured women to patient satisfaction surveys. Yet part of the reporting process for the Episcopal Health Charities was to determine if their funding "had an impact on the spiritual wellbeing of those served."

What a question. How on earth would anyone be able to measure spiritual impact or wellbeing? Most grantees avoided that question, after all it was optional, but I wondered what would happen if we simply asked our patients the question.

In today's world of evidence-based evaluations, that type of approach would never work, but back then we did a lot of things that would never meet the ideals of 'true research' standards.

My communications person created a beautiful one-page mailer. Its questions were encased with a fancy border, punctuated by a butterfly with its wings fully extended in the right hand corner of the page. The ten questions were typed in cursive font, and a translated Spanish version was included on the reserve side. The form was printed in two colors, volunteers helped label envelopes, stuff them, and in the mail they went.

The questions were basic: Were you treated with respect and dignity? Did you feel like your questions were answered? The last two questions addressed the task at hand: How did having a place to turn to for help impact your life spiritually? and What do you think is the connection between your physical health and your spiritual self?

In a million years, I could never have anticipated the number of returns or the different type of responses that we would receive. The willingness of women to share from their hearts, to talk about their faith, to recount their journey when all seemed lost at the point they were led to The Rose was profound.

I was impressed by the ability of these same women to so eloquently communicate their story. Spanish or English, all held a captivating quality, a very personal glimpse into someone's life. In fact, some of their answers were so personal I deliberately moved those pages out of the stack that would be copied for our funder.

But one response stopped me in my tracks, and it was one that did not come by return mail.

About three days after we sent the surveys, Dee barged into my office, her face was flushed, tears ran down her cheeks. "I have to tell you this," she said, her voice husky, breathless.

Now what? I wondered.

Whenever I came up with hare-brained schemes, her favorite saying was "It may <u>sound</u> good, but let's talk <u>real</u> world here."

Designing a special survey for our sponsored women was one of those schemes.

I smiled up at her, thinking that in spite of her 'let's get real' approach to life and an almost tough exterior, Dee was a softie and her tear-filled announcements weren't all that unusual.

"I just received a call from one of our sponsored women." She sat down in front of my desk, cocking her head to one side. "You will NOT believe what she said!"

Another set of tears welled up and poured through her eyelids. I reached for the box of tissues. Snapping one out, she dabbed at her face then continued, "This lady said there has been some mistake."

"Mistake?" I interrupted.

She nodded, "That's what she said, 'mistake.' The lady, her name was Clara, said, 'I got this letter in the mail from The Rose and you must have mistaken me for another patient.'"

Dee's wide open brown eyes grew even wider. "At first I thought she meant she wasn't sponsored," which was also the first thing that had jumped into my mind, "and so I asked her if she had insurance or had paid for her service.

"Clara, said, 'Oh no, I was helped by The Rose and I am so grateful for that. But this letter is much too pretty. It couldn't have been meant for me. I've never received anything this nice before.'"

My heart dropped.

Dee nodded, blew her nose, acknowledging the look on my face.

"That's right. That's what she said." Dee half-smiled, the tiniest catch in her voice. "It was too pretty for her to receive. I told her it was definitely meant for her and we would so much appreciate her answers and sending it back to us in the self-addressed envelope." As she repeated what she had said to the patient, Dee's voice was now warm and rich with authority. I was sure Clara would follow her instructions exactly.

She reached over, her hands covering mine, which were clasped together a little too tightly. "You were right, Dorothy. I'm glad we sent this survey—and made it look nice." She patted my hands and rose to leave, repeating, "Too pretty for her…" shaking her head as she left.

I remember sitting there, baffled. How could anyone, no matter how poor, really think that something was "too pretty" for them to receive?

Then the outrage hit me. *Too pretty?* I thought. *How could this be an issue for any woman? Had the divide between the rich and poor, hell, make that between the middle class and poor, become so wide that a person's worth could be reduced to whether or not she was 'worth' receiving something nice in the mail?*

How many times had I seen that lack of value demonstrated?

I'd seen it too many times in women we diagnosed at a late stage—that stage when the cancer was roaring through her body, eliminating most of her options and putting her life on the line. Almost without exception, that woman reluctantly admitted that she had put herself, her health, last on the list. Everyone and everything else was more important than her taking the time for an appointment. Oh, there would be a long list of other barriers that kept her from tending to that lump in her breast, the one she felt months ago, but hidden between every line on that list was the belief "I'm not worth it."

I've looked into the eyes of too many of those women, seen the fear and her inner knowing of what was ahead of her. I will never truly know how she feels. I can only watch her agony from a distance. The next phase of her journey will be hers alone. No amount of money or insurance coverage would make any difference at this point.

Then the sadness engulfed me. *What on earth could be going on in this woman's life that a simple letter decorated with a drawing of a butterfly would be the prettiest thing she had received?* I thought. *How could the world have become so bleak, life so difficult for her? This human being was someone we had served. How little we knew about her. How could we ever understand her sorrow, this person who didn't think she deserved a simple piece of paper?*

I remember touching my chest, as if I could console my heart, cover the hole that had opened inside of it, from the outside.

It was one of the days when those invisible hands on my shoulder shook hard.

Chapter 21
Pink Goats and Skydiving

Throughout the years, The Rose has received more than its share of gifts from uninsured women who want to give back. Sometimes it was donations of baked goods for the Shrimp Boil, sometimes they helped stuff envelopes for a mailing, but seldom did they bring cash. The first time it happened I couldn't believe it, but then the woman who brought it was pretty unbelievable.

Nadi was in her mid-fifties and lived in a tiny trailer somewhere out on County Road 937. She did odd jobs to stay alive but the oddest involved her climbing through brushes, over swampy wetlands, and sometimes up into trees to rescue baby birds driven from their nests by utility workers repairing lines. I never quite understood how she turned what was a very humane reaction to the birds' plight into a paying venture, but she did. The electric company paid her, albeit a pittance, for each bird she rescued and was able to keep alive. That meant hand feeding them for weeks, keeping them in her homemade incubator, and more times than not, burying the little ones who couldn't make it.

Almost a year after her biopsy, Nadi walked into The Rose, dressed as usual in her overalls covered in the evidence of her life, dirt stained, faded but nonetheless wearable. Her hair was long, unkempt; her lined face was sunburned but her nearly toothless smile was so genuine, she was beautiful. That day she was beaming with pride over the money she had raised.

"That should put a dent in my bill," she said as she handed Dixie an envelope filled with $952.

Dixie hugged her and said, "But you don't have a bill, Nadi, remember? The Rose sponsored your services."

"I know, but I figured that all you did for me cost a lot more money than that." She smiled up at Dixie, "I wanted to be sure you have some left for the next woman who might need it."

I forget now the number of nests or birds that were involved for her to raise that much money, but I do remember her saying, "You need to understand that I had to use some of the money I get for those babies, I need something to live on," she confided, sounding almost apologetic, "but I put a bit back from each nest...to bring to you."

Amazed at her sacrifice, I thought, *She might as well have brought us $9 million.* There was no way to put a dollar value on her donation.

The giving back continued throughout the years.

Ever since we started accepting insurance, The Rose has offered a cash discounted price for services. It was one of the ways we stayed true to our mission—and for some women, it meant their life.

At least that is what Judy will tell you.

"What would I want the world to know about The Rose?" Judy repeated my question. "If it had not been for The Rose's cash price, I wouldn't have kept up with my annual mammograms. It was fifteen years ago when I was diagnosed, and I still say it today. The Rose saved my life."

To Judy, it was that simple. "Remember, Dorothy, " her voice had a Texan accent, not the long drawn out words found in the people from East Texas, but that folksy, Southern hospitality cadence that lured one into another story. "Joe worked at one of the plants for thirty years; we never worried about insurance or healthcare. He had great benefits, we thought we were set." She was pretty, easy to look at, and must have been a knockout in her younger days. Today her makeup was perfect, her light, reddish colored hair stylishly coifed with a messy, fun quality to it. Fun was a good word to describe Judy. She had a way of finding humor in most everything, even when life was dark and scary and sad.

"When he lost his job, it was the first time in our married life when we didn't have insurance, but we were healthy and weren't worried. We opened that little neighborhood bar and made a living. It wasn't enough to purchase health insurance, but enough to live.

"We kept up with our annual examinations. One of my customers told me about The Rose. She said it was the lowest price in town, so I started coming to you. I never realized The Rose was a non-profit, in fact, I never knew you offered charity care—at least not until I was diagnosed. I had always paid my way, and I know a lot of other women who did also."

Judy had her annual mammogram, using our cash discounted program, for seven years. She teased me about the increase from $50 to $75 to $100 over those years, but she added, "It was worth it. I'll never forget the day I received that letter telling me I needed to come back in for another test. When it turned out to be cancer, I went into some kind of fog. I don't know what I would have done without The

Rose. That's when I found out you helped women who were diagnosed."

When Judy was diagnosed, we had barely started our navigation program and didn't have many resources. Thank goodness she had a family member who worked for a physician at Methodist and he was able to get her into their program.

"We got through the treatments, and I say 'we' because Joe was there with me every step of the way. I was so afraid. Everything was scary but the chemotherapy was the worst. I remember the first time I went in to have it. I was beside myself, I couldn't think, I was shaking all over. I didn't know what to expect. I had these visions of this burning stuff going into my arm and tearing up my insides." She paused, her face crumbled and tears filled up those big eyes of hers. "Joe took my hand and stroked my arm, and said, 'Honey, I would trade places with you…I would take that for you if I could.'

"Of course, we didn't know that a few years later it would be Joe having chemotherapy for his cancer," she sighed, her mouth trembling a little as she reached for the box of tissues on the table. "I had one of the good guys; that's for sure."

Joe had died five years ago and I knew Judy still ached for him; a person does that when she's been married to someone for 43 years, but more importantly, when that someone is a person who was truly loved.

Once Judy recovered from her treatments, she became our best ambassador, volunteering for TV and newspaper interviews. She had that 'woman next door' look to her and soon became our poster child, advocating for annual mammograms and early detection. She never really liked doing the interviews, but she told me, "If it could happen to me, then it could happen to anyone."

That was Judy's first 'giving back' to us.

Her next gift was raising money for The Rose—a lot of money. The first year she hosted Jamming for a Cause at her neighborhood bar, it raised $16,000! Next came dart tournaments, more jamming events, then she hopped on the Shrimp Boil committee. When we lost our cookers, she recruited Mark. He didn't just cook the shrimp but handled all the buying of the shrimp, potatoes, and corn, then secured the huge cooking pots and gathered his pals to cook the shrimp, all of it happening outside in the blazing July heat. He was also in charge of keeping the serving lines stocked, and each year made the flow better. He never missed a committee meeting and on the day of the event would show up at 9 a.m. and stay until 10 p.m.

Mark was one on a long list of people Judy led to The Rose; she was like one of those evangelists, recruiting anyone who expressed the slightest inclination to help. Her sister-in-law, Ella, created the eight by ten hand-sewn quilts that were the prized live auction item at the Shrimp Boil, one year bringing in $10,000! Her friend, Sharon, handled the dessert table and soon doubled the sales by encouraging more people to donate cakes and cookies. Judy's daughter, Jennifer, also helped out and had been part of our Bikers against Breast Cancer event since day one.

Judy's list of recruits was far reaching. But she insisted that the recruits she was most proud of were, "All the women I've told that they needed to have their mammograms done! Darn it!" She pounded the arm of her chair with her tiny fist. "Why, I didn't even know until last year that my story made Sharon go get her mammogram. And sure enough, she was diagnosed. I can't wait until I get to heaven, not only because I'll see Joe," her eyes sparkled as her smile widened, "but I'll also get to see all those other women who got to live a little longer because they listened when I told them to go get their mammograms."

Each year when we go through the process of creating the coming year's budget, I listen to the finance team argue about eliminating our cash discounted price for mammograms. That's when I remind them of Judy.

From birds to bars to bikers, the donations and giving back comes in all forms, but the most unusual has to be the Pink Goat.

I was in Canada when Palmer McInnis first made history with The Rose. Our board member, Bob Domec, had left a message on my phone, talking so fast I almost couldn't make out what he was saying. "Did you hear about the heifer? Palmer's heifer was covered in pink ribbons! The auction brought in $11,000!"

Heifer? Auction? Palmer who? I was totally confused and it was several hours before I learned the whole story.

The year was 2005. Palmer was sixteen years old and an avid FFA participant, having brought many animals to the Pasadena Livestock Show and Rodeo for showing and auction. That year, his stepmother, Carla, was losing her battle against breast cancer. Palmer's dad and stepmother ran their own company and times had been tough. They didn't have insurance, and when she needed help, The Rose was there.

Carla was in ICU when Palmer showed his prized heifer, and his decision to donate whatever money it brought during the auction to The Rose was pretty incredible. You have to understand that these young people usually apply their winnings to their college costs. In Palmer's mind, that money was better used by The Rose to help more women like his stepmother.

Fast forward one year later to the fall of 2006.

While I wasn't at the Livestock Show, I've heard many versions of the event—it was a once in a lifetime happening that will go down in history, not just for The Rose but also for the cities of Pasadena and Deer Park and most of all the Pasadena Rodeo and Livestock Show.

Carla had died not long after the donation from the heifer auction, and things got pretty tough for the McInnis family. His dad was in major grief, work was sparse and Palmer sure didn't have money to raise, feed, and care for another heifer. In fact, he didn't do a lot of things that his buddies were doing during their senior year.

Palmer is an incredibly handsome young man, with a modest 'aw shucks' approach to life and 'it was nothing' response to any praise. It is his sweet and generous nature that sets him apart. So that year he decided he couldn't give up. He raised a goat. A plain simple goat he named Poncho, and on the day of the Livestock Show, he spray painted the goat a bright pink color! (Folks asked if the paint hurt the goat—the answer was no, it washed off easily.)

His was an eighth place goat, not even in the running for any top awards and certainly not a candidate for earning much money from the auction. In fact, if it brought $1,000 it would be lucky. But, undaunted, Palmer put a big pink ribbon around that little goat's neck and pulled his pink package into the ring. He announced that whatever he raised from the auction would go to The Rose.

The auctioneer knew Palmer's story, his family's loss, and his wish to donate his winnings. Our board member, Bob, made sure the auctioneer knew that Palmer's heifer had raised $11,000 the previous year. Before the auctioneer called for the first bid, he shared the amount and Palmer's story.

Joe and Debbie, owners of an auto parts place in Pasadena, started the bidding off at $11,000! Everyone was stunned. A hush went over the arena. Then the bidding began. The total began to climb and in moments it reached $50,000, another bid from Joe and Debbie. At that point, Bob approached the auctioneer and told him Palmer's dad had raised another $10,000 to add to the pot and Casa Ole' was donating an additional $5,000.

The auctioneer made the announcement and that's when pure chaos entered the arena.

Someone else shouted, "I'll add $5,000!"

Another yelled, "Make that $10,000!"

In seconds, the crowd was going wild, clapping and screaming as one amount after another was offered, the frenzy was incredible. The auctioneer called for a stop to the bidding.

His attempt to stop it went unheeded, the crowd continued to raise the amount again and again and again.

The final figure came to $115,000.

Everyone was screaming and hugging. Folks were there from The

Rose, board members and employees—all of them jumping up and down. Brahana told me that she looked out over the crowd and saw grown men—real cowboys in their boots and hats—openly crying.

It was a moment never before experienced at the Pasadena Livestock Show, and most likely will never be recreated. Palmer's story was picked up by every news station and he was interviewed over and over by the local media. His answer to "Why would you do this, why would you give up your college money and be so generous to The Rose?" was always the same.

He'd smile and say, "It was the right thing to do. All those women at The Rose need help."

In the following months, we leveraged the excitement by starting the Pink Goat Society. For only $1,000, anyone could be a Pink Goat. For the next eighteen months, the Society was a mainstay for individual donations, moving our $1,000 givers from thirteen to eighty. What a difference this young man made when he decided to do something special in memory of a woman who meant a lot to him. Poncho eventually went to Dixie's ranch, where he lived out his short but famous life.

Most folks who give back have their feet on the ground. Not so with our most recent donor. She turned her event into an annual fundraiser and it became its own non-profit: Jump For The Rose.

Marian was in her mid-fifties, and although she had been successful in her own right, she abandoned her career path when she married. She and her husband enjoyed a comfortable life for many years, then, as life would have it, she awoke one day to find he had left and she was alone, broke and uninsured. Able to work as a manicurist, Marian was putting her life back together, or at least trying to, when she heard about a free mammogram screening program and signed up.

"That was the start of my journey with The Rose," she said. Marian sat across from me in the conference room. Ten of us had gathered to meet with her, employees from development, administration, accounting, and me. Marian had requested a time to make her presentation and take pictures, so we turned it into an impromptu reception with cookies, coffee, and soft drinks. Everyone was engaged by her story.

"When they told me I needed to have follow-up because they had found something on my mammogram, for some reason I really wasn't worried, even though my mother had breast cancer and a mastectomy at age fifty. When I had insurance I always had my annual mammograms—never missed it, it was what you did when you had a family history. But after the divorce, it had been a couple of years. One of my customers told me she was going to have a free mammogram through some program at the hospital. I jumped on it. I called and got the very last appointment they had. *Lucky me*, I thought.

"A week or so later they had me come back in and told me I needed an ultrasound and maybe a biopsy, they gave me a piece of paper that had two places listed on it, one was Harris County Hospital District and the other was The Rose. I had never heard of The Rose but the name sounded good. At least I imagined it would be better than Ben Taub, and besides, The Rose was closer to Baytown. I told them I'd go there."

Marian was tall, not skinny, not heavy, although she complained that the tamoxifen had put a few pounds on her. She was an avid skydiver, a hobby started in her former life that she still managed to enjoy now. Her physique was one of strength honed by activity, she moved effortlessly. She once told me that her skydiving gear was so expensive that she had to keep her weight in check; she sure couldn't afford to buy another suit.

Her cropped brown hair framed an open face, she had eyes that smiled and there was something bright and wholesome about Marian. Her voice was melodious, easy on the ears.

She shifted in the chair. "But by the time I was headed to The Rose for my appointment, I was starting to get worried. I really dreaded having to go to a charity clinic. I figured it would be some kind of storefront place in a strip center, much like the clinics I'd seen in Baytown, with lines of people waiting to be served. I hated the thought of going to a free clinic, one for poor people, but I didn't have any choice…" Her voice trailed off and she looked away, a memory of that worry and dread danced across her face.

She returned to her audience and continued, "Anyway, imagine my surprise when I drove up to this fabulous two story building and walked into that huge lobby area. Those marble floors were shining and everything was beautiful. I thought, *This can't be a clinic.* I still had that bad feeling, thinking that I would probably be grilled about my finances and why I didn't have insurance. I had never had to ask for any kind of help before. I felt so embarrassed—but I sucked it up. It was my life and I'd do whatever I had to. I brought all these papers and proof of income, but I figured I would face a huge hassle." She shrugged her shoulders.

My heart sort of skipped a beat. We worked hard to keep our process simple and smooth, but there was still a process and I feared her experience may not have been the best.

She continued, "I was so surprised. Everyone treated me so nice; I didn't feel like a charity case at all! It was like I wasn't any different from anyone else in the waiting room, like I belonged there, had insurance or whatever. I was amazed that I didn't feel like I was begging for help," she paused, her voice husky, "I was treated with dignity."

Her last words made tears spring to my eyes.

"But the best part, if having ultrasound tests could be called 'best,' was meeting Dr. Dixie. When she told me I would need a biopsy, I said, 'I don't know how I can have that done. I don't have any money.' Dixie patted my hand and told me not to worry about that part.

"I couldn't believe what she was saying, and asked, 'But how can you do that? How can you just give me a biopsy?' Dixie was so matter of fact. 'That's why I started this place,' she said, 'to take care of women like you.'

"After I had the biopsy and the cancer was diagnosed, I was really scared. But she said she would find me treatment, she had a navigator to help me and I didn't need to worry about anything except getting better. I kept asking her how she could get me into treatment. That's when Dixie told me how she got people to donate to The Rose, foundations and corporations.

"I remember looking up at her and saying, 'When I get better, I'm going to be one of those people who helps you—I'm going to raise a lot of money for you.'

"And that's why I'm here today!" She stood up. Her smile was almost as big as the huge white cardboard check she had created to use for the photograph. It proudly displayed the sum: $14,000! I gasped. I never expected it to be that much.

"I had hoped to raise more but..."

"Good gosh, Marian," I interrupted her, sputtering, "that is equal to...or more than...our grants!" I jumped up and went over to her, squeezing her tightly in a big hug, all the while babbling about what that meant to our program and thanking her. Watching Marian, I saw that familiar gleam of pride in her eyes, the same one I had seen in Nadi's, Judy's, and Palmer's.

I was again humbled by the effort, the concern for other human beings, most of all the plain ol' generosity that motivated people to give back.

By September, 2011, it was time for the second annual Jump for The Rose and Marian jokingly said, "You should come out and tandem jump with us, Dorothy."

"Actually, Marian, skydiving is on my list; one of my life goals."

She was so surprised. "Really? Then you must come out, we can plan a formation around your jump. It would be great publicity! I can't wait to call the team." She was off and running, talking a mile a minute about ideas, and out the door before I could stop her.

I hadn't agreed to do it, I had said it was a goal…one of those someday goals. But Marian had just turned someday into now.

By 7:30 a.m. on the day of the jump, I had signed in, watched the required video, and was being suited up. I tried to pay attention to Matt, the tandem instructor who would hold my life in his hands throughout the jump.

"After the door is opened, we will walk together to it. It's a little awkward but it's just a couple of steps." He led me to a mock-up of the cabin door and showed me how we would step out of the plane together. "Once outside, keep your knees bent, it helps with the free fall, at 6,000 feet I'll motion for you to pull the ripcord." He demonstrated his cues and reinforced how to pull the cord. "When we land, keep your feet and legs up; let me do all the work. That's all there is to it," he smiled.

Right, I thought.

Marian's cohorts surrounded me, giving me more last minute advice. "Keep your chin up and smile, otherwise all the video will capture is your cheeks flapping in the wind." Now that was the most important advice of the day!

"When I come up to you I'll grab your arm like this," Marian placed a hand on my forearm, "Don't jerk away, you may not see me until I'm right beside you. Leah will come up on your other side and do the same. The others will latch on and we'll stay in formation for a minute or so."

How could they do all that in a minute or so? I thought. I didn't know then how long a "minute or so" could be.

Soon I was struggling to climb up into a very small, very compact plane. As I reached the last step, I thought, *I'm 61 years old, what the heck am I doing?*

When we reached jump level, 14,000 feet in the air, the mood in the plane shifted. Everyone was serious, rechecking gear, and the chatter stopped. Matt motioned for me to move up next to him and locked me in. Someone opened the huge door at the side of the plane and a gust of wind filled the cabin.

It was time.

Matt sort of pushed and carried me as we frog-walked toward the door. I tried to remember the instructions but all I saw was the endless sky outside that gaping open door. We jumped. The noise of the wind was all-consuming. Free falling, traveling at 112 miles an hour, a human body plunging to earth for only a handful of seconds. Yet those seconds expanded to infinite time, filled up with every sense pitched to its maximum. A feeling of weightlessness conflicted with the sense of falling, the speed of moving through the rushing cold wind whipping around us, the sight of the land below, all forged together.

Suddenly someone was at my side, grabbing my arm, then another. Soon all the women were connected to each other and our formation was made. A person was falling right in front of us; it was the videographer filming every moment of our dive. I remembered to keep my knees bent, I remembered to smile.

I didn't remember to pull the cord when Matt signaled.

Snap! The harness jerked me upright, pulled hard against my crotch, and in less than a breath, we were floating. Hundreds of miles lay below; the sun still sat low in the eastern sky and the glow of dawn hued the earth with a golden color.

It took a few seconds to realize the sound of the wind was gone. All was silence, the earth, the sky, the water, if eternity could be captured in a moment, it was that one. I thanked God for the gift of seeing the world in its purest form, serene, beautiful, and unspoiled. Matt played with the lines of the parachute and soon we approached our landing. I didn't want it to end.

Back on the ground, all was celebration. With each hug, I felt my heart swell with such wonder, such gratitude for these men and women who challenged the sky for a cause.

Marian came up to me, a knowing look on her face. I couldn't quit laughing or talking. The surge of adrenaline would last for hours. She put an arm around my shoulder and said, "Now remember this, Dorothy. People are going to ask you, 'Why in the world would you jump out of a perfectly good airplane?' This is how we skydivers answer that question."

I looked up at her; my smile had become a permanent fixture on my face.

She leaned in and whispered, "You tell them, 'Because the door was open.'"

At The Rose, an open door means many things; most of all it means help for someone in need. Thank goodness for those people who show up at the most unexpected times with the most unexpected gifts and help us keep those doors open.

Chapter 22
Calling the Loan

Tom wanted to meet with me after the board meeting. The tone in his voice should have alerted me; after all, he had been on the board for nearly two decades. I had so much on my mind, I could barely concentrate, much less be sensitive to those subtle signals.

For over a year, I had gone to bed worrying and woken up worrying. Funding had been a constant challenge and for two years in a row, 2009 and 2010, we had had a deficit. Our fiscal year ran from August through July, and on this day in late January, 2011, we were already six months in. We faced the very real possibility of another year ending in deficit. There was no help in sight. The board had listened to the auditor's report: "Two years ago, raising the $2.3 million for equipment saved you. But last year and this year you spent that money on capital items—it's all listed here."

Ann distributed a spreadsheet, saying, "I realize that you'll start to see more revenue from having digital, but for now all of your reserves are used up."

She was correct; having digital would add $1.5 million annually in revenue, but that increase wouldn't be totally felt until next year. Converting to digital had taken way too long. The FDA approval process for the newer PlanMed system had been the culprit behind the delay. We had waited for over three years for that FDA approval on the digital equipment—three years of lost revenue!

The irony was that PlanMed had sold mammography systems in Europe for over fifteen years. In fact, we purchased all three of our mobile mammography units from them and never had one issue with any of their equipment. But mobile mammography units didn't threaten the big US corporations that made imaging systems and radiology equipment. Mobile units were small change.

The opposition came when PlanMed tried to introduce a reasonably priced yet equally excellent in quality digital imaging system in the US. We were stunned to hear that their digital equipment had to undergo a series of incredibly complex studies to satisfy the FDA, what should have taken a few months would turn into years. I don't have any proof, of course, but I have no doubt why it took so long. It wasn't the first time that the interest of the patient took a back seat to the interest of a company that had a lot to gain, or lose. It happens all the time in the pharmaceutical arena and healthcare devices; the list goes on and on. Everyone loses waiting on those approvals, everyone except the big guys.

But none of that mattered while we reviewed the audit. Every funding dollar had been used for equipment, which meant operational funding suffered severely. We were not in this boat alone. 2010 had been a tough fundraising year for many non-profits. Most folks blamed the struggling economy; most philanthropic foundations' portfolios since 2008 had declined. Funders weren't as amenable to large gifts and sure weren't maintaining their prior levels of giving. Over the past four years, annual gifts from our largest funder had dropped from $960,000 to the current amount of $450,000.

At least hiring Bernice as our COO was starting to pay off. She had spent months in negotiations with the VA, which owed us nearly a half a million dollars in back payments. Pam had won that account years ago, making The Rose the exclusive provider for VA mammograms. It was quite a coup for us and by far our largest contract, with the highest reimbursement per procedure. But the contract was up for renewal and there was lots of competition for it. We hesitated challenging their slow payments.

But not Bernice; she called in the Big Guns and laid out our case. We had to refile every single invoice and provide all kinds of documentation, hours of additional reworking on our part, but Bernice was a bulldog, she wouldn't give up. They continued to ignore her until she flatly refused to take any more of their patients unless they paid their bills.

No services for the female vets would have been a public relations nightmare for the VA, which was already making headlines about how long it took for any of their patients to receive care. It would take eleven long months, more meetings and a lot more refiling of claims before the balance was reduced to a reasonable amount.

Their tardiness was the reason for us having such a large accounts receivable, but I honestly wasn't aware of the alarm it generated with our bank until that day with Tom.

Tom is a handsome, small-boned man who stands an even six foot tall. He's the ultimate gentleman who always has an interesting story to tell, but that day his story was anything but funny. I studied him as he sat across from me, trying to focus on his words.

"I received a confidential call about our loan. The call was from a senior manager at the bank who is a friend of mine and knew I was on The Rose Board." Tom moved uneasily in the chair, looked down at his hands and steepled his fingertips. He looked back up at me. "There was a meeting yesterday at the bank that involved high risk loans. They have...uh...expressed concern about the financial ability of The Rose to meet its obligation with the loan."

High risk loans? I didn't understand. For the past year, we had provided the bank with monthly financials. Four months ago, Pam and I met with the new officer assigned to our account. I explained that we couldn't always gauge the timing of grant approvals. It was obvious that he never quite grasped that concept of grants but he assured us the meeting was routine, nothing to worry about.

Tom's words evoked a creepy feeling that started to spread through my body, making the hair on the back of my neck stand up.

"What does that mean, Tom? I know we've had two years of deficit..."

"It is not only that," he interrupted, flashing a half-smile my way, "although it is a factor and does have an impact and would have been much better if this past year had not been in a deficit. Actually, it has to do with debt ratios. When one looks at the debt to revenue ratio of The Rose, it makes it fall into the high risk category." He paused before continuing, "I believe the bank is not giving The Rose credit for all its income based on the nature of funds received...pending grants that are not a certainty, as an example."

He paused again, letting his words sink in. I was now cocooned in that creepy feeling. He shifted in his seat, shrugged his shoulders and pointed to an imaginary form on the table. "When that happens, a bank has the option of reducing its risk and moving the loan to an area of the bank that specializes in collections and liquidations. This would not be good for The Rose."

He looked at me; there was a question in his eyes. I shook my head still not understanding. He continued, "With the way they are calculating the debt ratio, not many banks would be in a position to hold our loan."

I flushed; the full meaning of his words slowly engulfed me. "What are you telling me, Tom? What exactly does all this mean?"

He looked back down, took a deep breath, the silence was palpable.

"Are you saying...are they going to call our loan?" I asked.

He nodded. My heart stopped.

"But how could they?" I tried to reason. "We've never missed a payment. We've never even been late on a payment."

"They can and it is a real possibility they will. If you read your contract with them, you'll see The Rose is in default based on ratios required to be maintained. There are a number of options the bank has which would allow them to take measures to reduce their risk."

"They could call the loan? And no other bank would want to take us on but they are the ones at risk?" My words were sharp, anger was rising.

"The problem is The Rose is not a large enough organization to be handled by the bank's not-for-profit division. In fact, the division of the bank that does handle our relationship is not that familiar with how a not-for-profit obtains adequate funding to support long term stability." He sounded weary. "Since grants aren't guaranteed, their top guys aren't going to even consider it as revenue. So, your debt ratio has fallen way below what your contract requires."

"But the grants ARE part of revenue!"

He nodded.

"We would never meet budgets with only the insurance or cash payments!" My voice had grown squeaky but it totally disappeared as I struggled with another question. "But what if we found a new funder..." The words were stuck in my throat and couldn't find a way out—exactly like I felt at that moment.

His voice was gentle. "They would find another reason to show the loan was in default. You don't understand, Dorothy. They don't care about The Rose. Sure, it could create some bad public relations for them, but that doesn't matter." His voice lowered, "They have all the power and they don't want our loan."

His words hung in the air. The room seemed to fade away, and at that moment, it was just me and Tom sitting in the middle of nowhere. He looked so chagrined I felt sorry for him.

This was the year of our twenty-fifth anniversary. We had fought so many battles, climbed over so many obstacles, and helped so many women. He was telling me that in the course of business, with a stroke of a pen, all those years could be erased. If they called the loan, we would lose The Rose. Images filled my mind, faces of employees, the women we served...a lifetime of work, the work of a lifetime...all gone.

After a few moments, I said quietly, "Tom, we can't make $2.6 million appear from nowhere. What options do we have?"

"With your permission, I want my folks to complete an audit on your books. I want to look at your financials from every perspective and apply our formula to it." He saw my face light up, but warned, "I'm not promising anything. Remember, every bank has to follow lending guidelines, and we only have so much latitude. The most important thing right now is to make sure I know if they call you for a meeting."

"They already have, Tom." My voice sounded dull, far away.

"When?" He genuinely looked surprised.

"Last week. Pam told me they called and wanted to schedule a meeting after the audit was final and had been discussed with the board. She was going to set it up for next week."

He thought a moment, pulled out his phone and was obviously tallying up days on the calendar. Something about this action made that sense of dread in me even more intense.

"I'll see if I can get our team in next week. I need to visit with Pam now." I nodded, he continued. "She'll need to pull a lot of information together for us to review. You'll have our best people."

"Tom, do you think your bank...is there any way...could take this loan?" I needed a crumb of reassurance.

"If it can be done, we will pay off the loan and move it to my bank." He nodded toward the door, "In the meantime, you and Bernice and Pam need to keep doing what you are doing. A few more months of being in the black will go a long way." He smiled, signaling our visit was over, always the gentleman, ending the meeting with a sense of graciousness and dignity. "Let us look over the books and I'll get back with you immediately." He put out his hand. His handshake was firm, his smile professional, but his eyes held no promise at all.

Chronic pain, much like chronic worry, can paralyze. One stops the body from functioning and the other stops the soul. And with nothing to stand on or lean against, the spirit crumbles. Both pain and worry had been my constant companion during those six months leading up to that day and the meeting with Tom.

I had a bad knee and it had steadily worsened until the pain was acute. After three years of trying every remedy, from over the counter pills, to Celebrex, to physical therapy, to two outpatient surgeries for meniscus repair and reaming out the arthritis, to injections every six months, I was more than crabby and walked with a definite limp.

My greatest nightmare was trying to walk up the stairs when the elevator wasn't working, which, during the past three years, was at least once every other month.

While the worry over finances and fundraising was going on, the daily pain in my knee had reached an unbearable point. My limp had gotten so bad that my right hand would drop, reaching mid-calf with each step. It was a sad sight. I couldn't wear heels and felt dowdy in my flats. The days of walking one to two miles each morning were long gone, and the weight was packing on. Simply put, I was pretty miserable.

After a bad fall during physical therapy, the therapist finally admitted, "You could consider having a knee replacement, but at 59 you're too young for that kind of surgery."

"What other option do I have??" I retorted, "Wait until I'm 65? I can't stay in this kind of pain even one more year, waiting another five years would be hell."

It wasn't just the pain; it was all the other hassles. With Patrick working overseas, meeting halfway for mini-vacations at exotic spots would have been fun. But I had to eliminate the most intriguing places because the tour information noted "walking" or "many steps" or "no elevator." Vacations aside, the daily compromises were impacting work. During a recent event to accept a check for The Rose, I had had to walk unassisted to the stage, down and back up a long aisle that was nothing but stairs. I don't know how, but I made it, teeth clenched and fighting back tears with every step.

So the search to find a knee surgeon began, and in August, 2010, I found the right guy.

"You have stage 4 disease," the surgeon said. "Your knee is bone on bone. I don't know how you are managing the pain now, especially without meds." He wanted to schedule the surgery immediately, but I needed to postpone it. "Why would you want to wait any longer?"

He obviously didn't realize that October was National Breast Health Awareness month or know about the number of presentations, events, and functions that I was required to attend. From the first week of September until mid-November, it was all about the pink: the Tour de Pink, the Komen Walk for a Cure, Cancer Fighters event, the list was long. This time of year was our high season, every weekend, three or four evenings each week, my presence was expected.

Dr. Lionburger shook his head as he left the exam room. I'd waited three years, what was two more months? I shrugged and took a deep breath while rubbing my sore knee, murmuring to it that soon it wouldn't hurt. I silently chided myself, *What are you whining about? What if this were cancer?* I had seen too many of our patients with metastasis to the bone. They were in real pain.

I hobbled out of the room, determined to make it through another few months without complaining. But the issues at work would soon take all the wind out of my sails. A perfect storm was brewing, and if something didn't change soon, the victims were sure to be our uninsured women.

While many non-profits have a large reserve or endowment to fall back on, The Rose started at zero each year and we didn't have many well-heeled folks in our back pockets to turn to during the lean times. Much of our financial issues were a result of the number of uninsured we served; over the past three years, that figure had skyrocketed, jumping from 4,000 a year to over 8,000. For fourteen months we handled the fallout of the devastation left behind by the 2008 storm, Hurricane Ike, which wiped out Galveston's Medical Center. It never occurred to us to turn those women away.

We had no sooner gotten out from under the deluge of the storm people, when we were faced with the thousands of people who had lost their jobs in 2008 and 2009 due to the decline in the economy.

We were so busy serving the unprecedented number of uninsured women, we totally missed the decline in the number of insured patients. The wait for our diagnostic appointments had reached four weeks. An insured woman needing an ultrasound or biopsy can go anywhere she wants for service and get an appointment a lot quicker than four weeks. For the uninsured woman needing those same services, The Rose was her only option.

But a bigger part of the decline in insured women was due to the fact that women were putting it off, afraid to take a day off work for a 'standard test.' That was a statement our schedulers heard often during the reminder calls to those women who were four, six months, or sometimes a year past due.

Even though it would not be apparent until late 2010, another part of the decline was due to the recommendations in November, 2009, from the US Prevention Services Task Force, which downgraded the recommendation level for mammograms for women aged 40 to 49. Once that report was caught by the media, with headlines screaming "Mammograms Harmful for Women," the annual screening rates across the nation took a nosedive. That was the fifth top story of 2009, and the results are a testimony to media's incredible power.

More than once, I would refer to the USPSTF findings as "idiot" recommendations. Most of the mammography community described it as a communications fiasco and the interpretation of the report as unfortunate. It was more than unfortunate—it was deadly. I remain convinced that that USPSTF recommendation alone carries the responsibility of women in their forties delaying having a mammogram and subsequently dealing with later stage cancers.

Studies have long supported the idea that it isn't 'cost effective' to screen younger women. Of course, if you or someone you love is one of those young women who become a death statistic, then studies don't matter much. An estimated 400 women in their forties would die each year if the 2009 recommendation were followed. That was not a number we could live with; we diagnosed too many young women.

But for all the 'statistical proof' the recommendations lauded, there was one fly in the ointment that no amount of scientific analysis could justify. One of the reasons for changing the recommendation was that mammograms supposedly "created undue anxiety in younger women who experienced more false positives and had to undergo additional testing or biopsies."

The statement about "undue anxiety" was clearly an opinion of the Task Force, not a fact supported by research. In all of my years of running The Rose, I have never met any woman who would rather skip having one extra test, especially if that test could confirm that she did not have cancer.

Unfortunately, following the USPSTF report, the number of women having annual screenings began to drop throughout the country, and has continued to remain at an all-time low. How tragic, since in September, 2010, the new healthcare reform required insurance companies to cover the cost of annual mammograms starting at age forty with no copay or no application of the cost to yearly deductibles, no out of pocket expenses, period.

The story of 100% coverage barely caught the media's attention. In fact, the only story I saw was a two sentence announcement buried under the government news section. No front page above-the-fold headlines to inform women of their 'new' coverage, which included annual pap smears, mammograms, and other preventative tests. (Sigh.)

Sometimes our troubles come from inside the organization, sometimes from outside, but when they come from both places at the same time it feels like walking through life bound by a straitjacket. One thing I knew was we needed help in a big way.

There was one foundation that we usually approached for larger needs, such as capital equipment, renovation, or relocating our second center. But the request we submitted in the Year of Worry was for operations. Pure and simple, we needed funding to continue. I had hoped for the best until I met with their grant officer. His responses were direct and discouraging.

"As I read your proposal, Dorothy," he leaned back in the chair, stretching out his hand, his fingertips touching the edge of the table, defining the distance between us, "you are asking the foundation to provide funding for the number of uninsured you expect to serve in the coming year." His tone was guarded.

"That's correct. As you can see, for the past five years the number has increased steadily, but it was nothing like the jump we've seen in these past two years."

"Dorothy, it seems to me that The Rose is in the same position as most non-profits, too many needing services and not enough funding. There will always be more people to serve, especially more uninsured." He shifted in the chair, uncrossing his legs, but the distance remained.

"There are too many organizations, like yours, trying to fill a need that can never be met."

I started to protest but he lifted his hand, palm toward me. "No," he continued, "the foundation wants to see outcomes, not more numbers. Our focus isn't the uninsured. Our focus is on what will strengthen the community as a whole."

My insides churned as I searched for a reply. My mind refused to function, thoughts revolved around my 'would be' responses like a needle caught at the end of the rings on the old-time 78 records. If this foundation didn't care about the poor we were lost.

"But the uninsured are part of the community, and when uninsured don't get care it creates another problem, a big problem..." I interjected.

"And that is why the foundation contributed, significantly," he interrupted and paused to let the last word sink in, "to a systematic approach of improving healthcare with its three-year commitment to the Alliance."

I knew about the $9 million grant, a collaboration of funding from the major foundations in an effort to increase primary care among the Federally Qualified Health Clinics in Houston. It was a pile of money and left out organizations like us.

"The Rose is the provider for mammography to all of those FQHCs! They don't offer that service, but you know they have to prove they have places to refer their patients to—it's part of their mandate and makes their government funding possible!" I pleaded. "Doesn't that make a difference?"

"Honestly, Dorothy. As I read the proposal I didn't see that you have a compelling argument for me to present to my trustees."

Compelling? The word stuck in my throat, but I croaked, "Eight thousand women, the population of a small town, that isn't compelling?"

"As I said, there will always be more uninsured. Perhaps the only solution is for The Rose to stop serving so many people." He sat back. "I realize you don't want to hear me say that, but the truth is, reducing the number of uninsured could be the only choice you have." The last words were sharp. He waited.

His words sunk in.

"You are absolutely right. I don't want to hear that." I leaned forward, trying to stay pleasant, but knowing the look in my eyes was anything but. "Tell me, how are we supposed to decide who we DO see? Which uninsured woman do we pick, who do we turn away? Should we be like public health and only accept fifty applications a day? Or do I decide that we only take those women who apply on

Monday, or whose last name starts with an S?"

"I didn't say that..." he started, but this time I interrupted.

"They all meet the criteria. We don't allow women who don't meet the criteria to have services. They are all eligible—every single one of them. How could we decide who gets help and who doesn't?" I honestly wanted an answer. It never came.

I tried a different approach. "If serving more uninsured won't make a difference, what would?"

"Find a way to be sustainable," he replied, almost too quickly. "We are encouraging every non-profit to attain, or at least try to reach, a level of sustainability so that they won't have to come to the philanthropic community year after year for funding." His words were measured. "You have a revenue stream, which means The Rose is better off than most agencies. The foundation might consider funding a business plan that would lead to sustainability."

No challenge there. The thoughts raced through my mind. *Continue to be a non-profit, provide uncompensated charity care to thousands of women, and become sustainable at the same time?*

After a few minutes of cautiously worded suggestions from him and clumsily worded inquiries from me, I agreed to go back and rewrite the proposal.

It came through loud and clear that The Rose was on extremely thin ice. This foundation was the pacesetter; all other funding organizations followed their lead. If the poor didn't matter to them anymore, then it wouldn't be long before we broke through to the icy waters below.

That afternoon, I was part of a video with nine of our sponsored women who had been diagnosed. Only one, Cindy, had been out of treatment long enough to have any hair at all. She had been in her early thirties when diagnosed; she held two part-time jobs to care for her two children. She remained up and optimistic even though she was dealing with a husband who left her after he couldn't handle her cancer.

Another one was Mary, who was so excited to have a really nice wig, styled just for her because she wanted to look pretty at her daughter's wedding the following week. Then there was Carol, a woman in her early sixties, who didn't have enough money for the gasoline to travel from Cleveland to the Medical Center for her treatment. She'd missed two chemotherapies before we found a small grant to cover transportation costs.

Our youngest was Melanie, who was diagnosed at 23 with stage 4 breast cancer, and would live with it and be in treatment for the rest of her short life. Then there was Tina, a pianist who recently played at one of our events. She had come to the video shoot immediately following chemotherapy, retching the entire way, because she didn't want to let us down. "After all," she explained, "The Rose has been there for me."

I didn't know Maria well but she greeted me with the biggest smile and I nodded to her and her daughter, Josie, who sat off to the side. Maria didn't speak English very well and didn't drive, so Josie was usually by her side.

Angela, a tall woman in her mid-fifties, didn't start with The Rose. She'd paid cash for her mammogram and ultrasound at a local hospital, but when she needed a biopsy there was no money left. Someone told her about The Rose.

The last two women were recently diagnosed and new to our support group. I hadn't met either yet. Soon I would learn of their journey, of how they found The Rose and how grateful they were to find help.

As the photographer instructed us to smile, I realized that all the camera could capture was a picture of women, different faces, different ages, and different races, most wearing scarves to hide bald heads.

The one thing the camera could never capture was their insurance status.

As I looked around at the women, I wondered, *Which one would we have picked? Who could we have turned away?*

Chapter 23
The Rescue

I hung up the phone. The conference call with the board was over. All morning, as I stumbled through employee orientation, I had dreaded making that call. By now every member of the board knew about the very real possibility that our loan was about to be called. It was the biggest challenge The Rose had ever faced.

I reported on the meeting with the grants officer and explained that we couldn't look to his foundation for help, at least not in the near future. We went over the financials and the cash flow projection again. Tom said his group was still looking at our books. I outlined the steps we were taking internally. Closing down the second center and eliminating mobile services were next on our agenda. We had sent updated profit and loss statements for both those areas to the board. Difficult questions were asked, different scenarios discussed, all between uncomfortable silences that seemed to last an eternity.

By the end of the call, the only decision that was made was for us to keep hanging on. I sighed and steeled myself for the next meeting.

"If we ever want to be funded again, there is no way we can have another year showing a deficit." I sat at the head of the table in our conference room. To my left and my right sat the five people who held the most responsibility in our organization, my executive team. They were responsible, I was accountable. The difference is equal to the chasm of the Grand Canyon.

The women around the table were unusually quiet. They all knew the trouble we were in, and even I was struggling to comprehend the depth of it. In the past, we had always managed to get by, some fundraising event would shower money on us or some grant would come in and save the day. Most likely that wouldn't happen this time.

We knew exactly which grants would come in, and the only big event between now and the end of July was the Shrimp Boil. If we worked real hard, we might net $60,000. That was a far cry from covering the $500,000 Pam projected we would need to break even.

The group squirmed, not only because of the conversation, but because those donated chairs were so darn uncomfortable. The hydraulic mechanism to lower or raise the seats had ceased to work long ago and they were all at different heights. Today Brahana, the tallest of our group, sat in one of the lower chairs, her chin dangerously close to the table, while Amy, our shortest, sat in a taller one, her feet not touching the floor, and reminding me of the Queen of Hearts on her throne.

I shook my head, trying to refocus. After so many sleepless nights, the days were foggy, but what was I thinking? Queen of Hearts? Had I fallen into the rabbit hole? Would a creature jump out from the closet, announcing, "You're late! You're late!"

It was late, very late in the game for The Rose. I shook my head again.

Bernice's voice broke the silence. We had a plan, but even if we were successful, it wouldn't be enough. "We are cutting every possible expense," she said, distributing a list of items we were eliminating. It ranged from sending back all the Ozarka water stations to cutting out the lump sum amount we annually provided to the employees' 401(k) plan.

"Effective March 1, tomorrow, there is a hiring freeze and no open positions will be replaced. If someone leaves, we will just have to work around it." Folks stirred. Bernice continued, "No raises, no matter who it is. No overtime. And," she took a breath, "we are cutting hours for everyone—32 hours a week for most. Unfortunately, the group that will be most impacted will be mobile." She glanced at Amy.

Even though I knew it was a necessity, I argued with Bernice about the plan to cut back mobile visits that served uninsured sites.

"You don't understand, Bernice," I explained, handing her my latest configuration showing every funder who provided money for sponsored procedures. "If we cut all sponsorship, we won't be able to meet the goals in these grants. Don't you see? If our numbers aren't close to what we projected, we won't receive the second part of the funding."

She sighed, "So we get caught either way?"

I nodded.

"But Dorothy, none of these grants cover our cost, even the Medicare rate doesn't come close!"

The actual cost of doing a mammogram was nearly $200. Providing sponsorship to the uninsured required using more resources. To top it off, we offered a cash discounted rate of $100 to make mammograms accessible to all, losing money on those exams.

Hospitals offer a 'loss leader' service like mammography because they have downstream revenue from lab, x-rays, and surgeries. The reimbursement involved in providing radiation therapy alone could make up for all the losses mammography incurred.

But The Rose didn't have downstream resources, and we did not provide those big bucks procedures such as MRIs or CAT scans. There wasn't a downstream for us, and as a result we were always swimming against the current.

"The other thing we will have to do is start asking for a copay from every sponsored women." Bernice distributed another piece of paper listing the different amounts for copays according to the cost of each service, $40 for a mammogram, $150 for an ultrasound and diagnostic mammogram, $300 for a biopsy.

"But we have always asked sponsored women if they can pay anything against their bill," Brahana offered.

"It's not near enough," Bernice said, shutting that argument down immediately, or so she thought.

"How can we do that? Most of these women don't have any money," Amy demanded, ending the silent spell from her end of the table, her voice was hot with anger. "Once again, it is the ones who need the most, the poorest, that will get penalized!" She spat those words out and glared at me. "I don't like that idea at all."

"It isn't a matter of us liking the idea, Amy," I started to explain. "The hardest sell we are going to have is with our employees."

Heads nodded.

Bernice sighed. "You're right. It won't be easy for our employees to ask uninsured women for copays, they have a hard enough time doing that with insured people." Her comment wasn't missed by anyone. "No matter how much we explain this change is needed, it's a cultural thing. Our employees identify with the uninsured. It will be hard for them."

There was more discussion; one argued they simply had to replace a position. "No exceptions," Bernice responded firmly, "even Dorothy can't hire an assistant now."

I met with Bernice afterwards. She was a savvy business person with decades of experience in healthcare. She had been part of the upper echelon at Baylor, reporting to the top gun and managing clinical responsibilities with a budget exceeding $100 million.

She left Baylor when the pressures threatened to destroy her health. She officially retired and took a year off from the craziness.

When the recruiter found her, Bernice was rested, bored, and ready to return to work. The one criteria she had for going back to work was that whatever job she found, it had to be meaningful, whatever she did in this last phase of her career had to make a difference in life.

She stood about five foot nine and usually dressed in conservative pinstripe pant suits. Brown was a good color on her, bringing out the copper in her brunette hair and lighting up her clear blue eyes. She was only four years younger than me but her cheery "Good morning!" announced her "It's a new day!" attitude, which made her feel a lot younger.

Today, that cheery attitude had gone on vacation.

There had been many times when The Rose struggled to maintain a positive cash flow, but only one other time that was this dire. That was the time when I planned to withdraw my retirement to cover payroll. Unfortunately, those funds wouldn't make a dent in fixing the financial dilemma we were in this time, and sure would not impress the bank.

As I left her office, I looked back over my shoulder at Bernice. She had slumped back in her chair and sat motionless with her gaze fixed on the wall facing her desk.

We're up against a wall, all right, I thought. *And I don't know how we'll get over it.*

There is a scene in the movie *Starman* where the creature from outer space is talking to Sherman, the government agent who has been hunting him down, and finally has Starman, exhausted and near death, trapped. Drawing upon his last bit of strength, Starman tells the agent, "You earthlings are a strange species. Not like any other. And you'd be surprised how many there are. Intelligent but savage. Shall I tell you what we find most beautiful about you?" Sherman nods. Starman says, "You are at your very best when things are the worst."

No other phrase could better describe my employees during those awful months from March through July in 2011. We held regular town hall meetings with small groups of employees. We shared the pending fiscal dilemma and explained our strategies. But the words that announced the hiring freeze, eliminated any merit raises, and talk of the reduction in work hours hung in the air. I looked into the faces of the people who really made The Rose run. There were some oldies wise to our history with all its ups and downs, but most were new.

We initiated the reduced hours. Most people exhausted their paid time off balances and were left having to be off work without pay. Counting on 40 hours a week and seeing it drop to 32, then 28, then 20 was difficult. One employee's husband had been out of work for over two years and she faced losing her home. Another employee was the sole support of three grandchildren. Our organization had more than its share of single mothers, caring for kids and living paycheck to paycheck. Even so, very few people left our employment during that time, the majority hung in there.

During those town hall meetings, seeing my employees' eyes wide with fear, I could not let them see the implosion happening in my gut. The world was falling in on me, it sure wasn't a perfect world, but it was the only world I had known for over 25 years.

In the business world, a widget is worth 'X' amount of money and the better the widget or the more you sell directly correlates with how well the staff is paid. Yet no matter how many appointments or work-ins or exceptional efforts were accomplished, my employees still made the same amount of money.

Our sponsorship coordinator, Elizabeth, came to me with a plan. "Dorothy, what if we got some people to donate cases of soft drinks and bottles of water. Instead of us putting money into the vending machine downstairs, we charge fifty cents for each. I bet we could raise enough to cover a few mammograms!" Her smile was bright.

We had put a limit on sponsoring basic screening mammograms so that we would have enough money to cover diagnostic work-ups. Elizabeth knew those tests could easily mean a woman's life. As she had many times before throughout her ten years of working for us, she was looking for another way to get her job done and serve those women needing help.

Our austerity measures had been in place for three months, and each month we managed to be a few thousand dollars ahead. But no additional funding had come in. We were far from out of the woods and our cutbacks were taking a different kind of toll. The mobile mammography staff was hit the hardest by the reduction in work hours. So many of our mobile sites served the uninsured, and with less funding we could no longer carry the sites.

Every week I was telling one community partner after another that we simply could not cover the costs of our mobile units going to their clinics any longer. Their women would have to wait until after July, and even then there were no promises. One clinic director came to meet with us. We had served her clients for seven years and had diagnosed over twenty women. Her clinic served the poorest of the poor. "Surely there is some way you could continue to come to our clinic," she pleaded, but our answer was no. God, I hated letting her down almost as much as I hated asking our employees to take days off without pay.

After that meeting, by the time I walked the short distance from the conference room to my office, I had worked up a ton of mad—at the bank, the world, the situation. I shut my door soundly, just shy of a slam. I looked around the room. I wanted to throw something, break something, anything!

After three years of just getting by, two of those in deficits, everyone was tired. It was more than the garden variety kind of tired; it was a weariness that went to the bones. *Could the bank really 'call' the loan?* I ticked off the facts in my mind. *They don't consider grants to be revenue. How insane. We are a non-profit, for crying out loud!*

Images flooded my mind: foreclosure signs hanging from the front doors; employees leaving in tears with their belongings in boxes; our hard earned and fought for and incredibly expensive equipment sold at auction for a pittance; the furnishings, chairs, pictures, bookcases, desks all lovingly donated, now tossed into a giant heap in a dumpster.

I shuddered at the next image, cold sweat poured over me. Patients were coming up the steps to the building, young women, old women, some exhausted from a long bus trip, finding padlocks on the doors. I watched them turn away and slowly descend down the steps, knowing some would die.

I cringed at the image of our sign being torn from the building. The Rose was no more. One picture after another clicked in my head, all doom and gloom, creating a PowerPoint of the pending demise of The Rose. I held my head in both hands, shut my eyes, trying to force the images away.

"Stop it!" I said aloud. "Stop it now!" I said again, my voice edged with anger.

I didn't hear the knock on the door but suddenly became aware that someone was near me. Startled, I opened my eyes, staring at the person standing in front of my desk. It was my manager over the Development Department. Pure terror covered her face.

"Here's the file we talked about...the Cullen Trust for Health Care," she said hesitantly, setting a folder down on my desk. "Are you all right? Do you need anything else?"

No, I shook my head, thinking, *I need a lot of things, but right now I need the right words and someone willing to listen to us. Someone who cares about the poor.*

The Cullen Trust was one of the few foundations that might consider an emergency funding request.

I picked up the phone. The first ring echoed in my head. My heart was beating so fast my chest hurt, and was so loud I was certain it would be heard over the telephone line. Another ring. I almost hoped no one would answer.

"Hello. This is Carol." The familiar voice tinged in a Northeastern accent came across the line. Carol was a consultant to Cullen Trust, she was the person who visited sites and vetted the proposals before they went to the trustees. She was legendary in the non-profit arena and one of the most exacting researchers I'd ever met. No nonsense, keen in finances, her method of probing was frankly intimidating and much like Barbara Walters, she asked those unexpected questions that people felt compelled to answer. Once she had asked my front desk staff if they thought I did a good job as CEO. Poor things, they didn't know what to say.

Actually, I admired her deeply. Over the years, after many site visits and discussions about our proposals, I had grown to really like her. Her dry wit and humor usually made me laugh.

For whatever reason, on this day, her voice was especially kind. I don't remember what I said to her, my well planned speech evaporated the moment I heard her voice. I do remember her replying, "You need to call Beth directly." It was a short conversation, matter of fact and to the point, as only this lady could be.

I took a deep breath, picked the receiver back up and dialed another number. Steeling myself, I made the call to the President of the Cullen Trust for Health Care, Beth Robertson.

Outsiders often think non-profits should operate with volunteer staff. They don't understand that it takes a highly trained technical staff to pass the FDA inspections each year and that physicians expect to be compensated for their work. Thank goodness, Beth understood. Her family's foundation had built much of the Medical Center and local universities. The Cullen name topped the list in philanthropy and the Trust that was devoted to healthcare had truly made significant changes in healthcare systems. They understood the need for operation funding if programs were going to function.

It seemed to take forever to finally talk with Beth, but actually it was only three days. She was away on vacation, yet her staff realized the urgency of my call and reached out to her. (I've added her assistant to the Band of Angels who walked alongside us during that time.)

While I didn't know Beth well, I had once served with her on a strategic planning committee for a community project. She was a petite woman and a natural beauty, her dress was almost casual, nothing showy but always fashionably classic. I remember watching her maneuver through those meetings with her banker's mind, keen on the bottom line and cutting through any fluff. Most of all, she was gracious. This was a woman of style and confidence, who understood that her role and influence in the community extended beyond her wealth.

"What's going on, Dorothy?" Her opening question went straight to the reason for my call. No chit chat, no small talk.

I described the situation, our 'perfect storm,' briefly alluding to the problem with the bank. I explained how encouraged we were by having five months in a row with revenue outpacing expenses (primarily because of the higher reimbursement for digital) and detailed the cost-cutting efforts underway to hedge against the next three months. But no matter what, despite the increased revenue, despite the cost-cutting efforts, by fiscal year end we projected being in the hole. I thanked her for their past funding and said that I realized any consideration to a request now would be a grant given outside their usual guidelines.

"What would it take for you not to end the year with a deficit? How much money do you need?" Again, her direct manner caught me off-guard. I was expecting she would need a lot more information before I reached the dollars point.

"$300,000," I squeaked. I cleared my throat and repeated, "We are confident that $300,000 would allow us to end the year in good stead."

"Dorothy, you may not know it, but we have finished our grant cycle for the year. The trustees are now on vacation, they have all gone away for the summer. The next meeting to review proposals isn't scheduled until September."

I bowed my head, holding it with one hand, willing the fingers of my other hand to hold the phone firmly in spite of its shaking. She had been my last hope. I felt a sharp pain in my chest and was startled by its intensity. Was I having a heart attack? Or was it caused by my oxygen-starved lungs screaming for relief from holding my breath?

"But I know how to find them. Let me see," she paused, "there is one who just left the country, so it may be a little difficult to reach him. It will take at least a week, maybe more, to talk with all of them and to send the information to them. Here's what I want you to do..."

She began to list all the documents she needed, everything she would want to share with her trustees. "You do realize that I can't approve this kind of request by myself. I have to have everyone agree to it. Could you send this information to me, via email, in the next day or so?" she asked.

I nodded my head.

"Dorothy? Are you there?" Her voice was sharp, and I realized I had gone dumb with wonder. She was actually going to consider it. I knew it wasn't a done deal yet, but she was actually willing to consider the emergency grant. It was a miracle.

"Yes, Beth. I'm here," I choked, hearing the tears starting from way back in the depth of my throat, knowing that she had heard them also. "I'll have it all ready for you today."

I worked late that Thursday evening getting everything together for her. It was a little past 7 p.m. and I had been at my desk since 7 that morning. All day long, huge storms had moved through Houston and the dark clouds matched my mood.

About that time, Tresa appeared at my door, her hair was plastered down and her words tumbled over each other. "I have to tell you a story. Do you have time?"

I nodded.

"We were out today at South Health Clinic and all the patients were late, they waited until that horrible weather came through so we ran behind. It was raining like crazy when we were loading the equipment. I'm grumbling and starting to feel sorry for myself when a car slows down, stops, and this woman got out. She was wearing old clothes, almost rags, and had a cap on her head. I was a little afraid watching her come running up to me, but then the woman said, 'You are with The Rose?' I said yes. Then she said, 'I thought so when I saw the van. I had to tell you that last year The Rose came to my church and found my breast cancer. I didn't have any insurance, and when the mobile unit came I felt so lucky to get to have a mammogram. When the cancer was found, you took care of me. The Rose got me into treatment.'"

At this point, Tresa's face grew solemn. "I thought, *What do I care about rain or getting wet? This lady, who is obviously having chemotherapy, stopped and got out of her car—in the middle of the rain—just to tell us thank you!*"

She smiled and turned to leave. "Can you imagine, Dorothy? That woman, with her hair all gone, with all she has to live with, was thanking me...for finding her cancer. When she touched my arm, I realized that no matter what kind of problems I have, no matter that I don't have enough hours, nothing I'm going through can compare to what she is dealing with."

She looked at me, her eyes alive and piercing. "When things like this happen, that's when I know why I do what I do. And no matter what, The Rose has to go on."

And the staff did just that—kept going on. The daily sacrifices continued. During all those long months, heaviness walked the halls. It greeted us at the doors as we entered, cascading worry upon our heads. It followed behind us with each decision. By the day's end, it had exhausted us with its relentless pummeling. But our defiance was tangible.

It was the employees who turned July's annual Shrimp Boil fundraiser into the most successful one in over twenty years. They donated items for the auctions, they coerced friends and family to purchase tickets, and in the end it raised just over $80,000.

Throughout all the town hall meetings, the staff's overriding concern was if they'd have a job. Every hospital and medical center in town was laying people off. Why would The Rose be any different?

My one promise to the employees was that they would have a job. They would not have all the hours they wanted, but they would have a job. It was a promise that I repeated at every gathering and included in every update email to staff. I had absolutely nothing to back up that statement, but somehow I knew it would be true.

And it was.

It all came together: Beth's board of trustees approved the emergency grant (it turned out to be only the second one in their history); the employees and their gifts of working less and giving more kept expenses in check; even the sponsored patients stepped up to help by paying what they could—no matter how small the amount—it all added up. We ended the year in the black.

That positive bottom line opened the doors for other possibilities. Within a month, our loan was taken over by Tom's bank, at a much better interest rate, without a balloon payment hanging over us and with a group who understood non-profits. The better financial standing also opened a line of credit, which meant that, if needed, we could purchase equipment without waiting for a grant. Most of all, ending the fiscal year in the black provided the success that was needed to approach other foundations with requests.

On a hot and muggy Monday morning, I was standing in front of the Kroger's grocery store waiting for it to open. Once inside, I purchased every rose they had in the florist section, filling up two grocery carts. Thank goodness they had a sale going on because the cost was out of my pocket. Even if they hadn't, I was determined to make this a special day.

I hauled my load of flowers, along with the vases I had scrounged from home, into our building and up the stairs to our kitchen area. For the next hour, still too early for most folks to arrive, I snipped off stems, plopped the flowers in vases, and lined up one arrangement after another on the conference room table. I was checking off my list when Bernice came in the room.

"What are you doing?" she asked, eyeing the mess of leaves and stem ends covering the counter top and trash cans overflowing with plastic bags.

"It's August 1!" I announced.

"Yes…and…?" she said slowly.

"And, we made it!" I exclaimed. I glanced through the door at the filled vases sitting on the conference table and smiled. "Help me take these to the different departments! These are a thank you to them. There is a name on each vase. As soon as I finish here I'm headed to the other center!"

We had made it. Months later, the annual audit would confirm what I knew that day; we had ended our fiscal year without a deficit.

We learned a lot from that difficult time—important lessons and a few facts that were hard to swallow. I had to come to grips with the reality that no matter how many services we provided, no matter who we served, no matter how much good work was being done within our walls, our very existence depended on the good graces and generosity of other human beings. I also had to acknowledge that some of those humans had no clue about The Rose's impact and really didn't care about the poor.

Yet people like Beth, and the foundations that women and men like her represent, understood at a profound level.

As we stumbled into the new fiscal year, still watching every penny spent, I sighed in relief that we had made it through the worst year of The Rose's existence. I had no idea what was lying ahead of us. The next year brought a whole new meaning to the word 'worst.'

Chapter 24
The Other Side of the Mountain

I was accepted as a fellow in the American Leadership Forum in January, 2011, and I looked forward to every meeting. The 26 CEO and top management men and women in my class were a diverse bunch with years of experience in business and non-profits. All of us had made a fifteen month commitment to ALF, agreeing to meet monthly, attending an occasional two day retreat, and sharing a week-long Wilderness Experience in Colorado.

For one day each month, I gave myself permission to leave the problems of The Rose and the worry over the loan behind. There was so much to learn from the group. The ALF's focus was different from any other leadership training I had ever taken; each meeting was mind-opening and innovative. I drank in those times like a thirsty nomad stumbling onto an oasis.

Going on the Wilderness Experience had been talked about since our very first meeting. But nothing prepared me for the physical toll of hiking to the top of a 10,000 foot high mountain peak on that day in mid-June.

"Let me carry your backpack," Karun offered, his deep voice sing song and pleasant. He was the clown of the group, his sense of humor always brought a laugh but at this moment he was totally serious.

I politely declined, silently affirming to myself that I would carry my own pack. Those 25 pounds were mine to carry, that was part of the deal, and each of us knew that we would be carrying a backpack going in to this hike. I was going to be equal to the others.

"Look," he pointed to a couple of other classmates, "Art is carrying Michele's."

I glanced over at my classmate; we were about the same age. She was moving easily now without the extra weight, her steps confident, her laugher animated and free.

No, I shook my head, and said, "I'll be okay."

He smiled, "If you change your mind, I'll be nearby."

Before the hike, the bulk of our days and nights during that week had been spent in the throes of nature, exploring the extent of our endurance and rediscovering the entity of self. I was next to the oldest person, Mel was three weeks older but he was in much better shape than me, as were eighty percent of the other men and women trudging alongside me up the rocky, steep hillside.

None of them had a knee replacement six months ago, I grumbled, trying to assuage myself. In spite of training for this trip, walking three miles a day in those horrendous hiking boots for two months and working with weights for upper body strength, I was definitely struggling. In fact, the whole past week had danced between struggle and adventure.

We were in the wilderness; that was certain. Cell phones were not allowed and internet services were non-existent in this remote area of the Pike National Forest in Colorado. For six days and nights, the simple things we took for granted—a diet coke, a glass of wine, or a bathroom of our own—didn't exist. Even breathing was a luxury at this high level and a couple of classmates struggled with altitude sickness. At least the women's dormitory and sleeping quarters were inside the main building; the poor guys had a choice between unheated, exposed to the elements yurts or an equally cold cabin with multiple bunk beds.

The Bison Peak Lodge offered a large open design, with the kitchen on one side and a huge fireplace on the opposite wall. A large community meeting area was filled with tables, chairs, and couches. Its wide, welcoming porch was lined with rocking chairs and looked out over an incredible view of the mountainside. Behind the Lodge was a huge fire pit trimmed by stone ledges.

Each person was assigned a 'buddy' and had their own 'sounding board,' a small group of six to eight people. The first four days were spent adapting to communal living, eating and completing exercises designed to build trust in one another. A walk along an uneven ledge while blindfolded was scary enough, as your buddy became your eyes but could guide you only with a touch of his or her hands, words were not allowed. Another exercise had a person standing in the middle of their sounding board partners and falling backwards, confident no one would let him or her fall completely to the ground.

The Power Shuffle or Crossing the Line exercise was intense, exposing those hidden places in a person's life and leaving no one—if they fully participated—untouched.

"Each person needs to respond to the question as he or she understands it," the facilitator stated.

All 26 of us stood in a line behind a long, wide red ribbon on the ground. Twenty feet away, running parallel to the first one, was another red ribbon.

The questions began, "Were you ever hungry and didn't know where your next meal was coming from?" The group shifted as the question sank in.

"If so, please cross over to the other side of the line." The facilitator waited as a handful of people hesitantly walked across to the opposite ribbon; then she continued, "Notice who is with you and who is not with you."

The handful of folks looked at each other and then, almost as a group, looked across to those standing behind the original red ribbon.

"Now return." The final instruction brought a sense of relief as those of us who had crossed over rejoined our friends.

The questions continued, one by one, measured in the asking, an eternity passed in the answering.

"Were you ever a single parent?"

"Did you ever lie about your age to get a job?"

"Have you ever worried about walking down any street in America with your significant other?"

"Were you poor?"

"Were you ever abused or watched a person you love be abused?"

Each question was followed by the mantra, "If so, please cross to the other side. Notice who is with you and who is not."

As a group, we shuffled through each question, sometimes the majority would cross to the other side.

"Do you have an advanced degree or certification in your field?" Yes, the majority answered, as most of the bodies moved to the other side.

Sometimes only two or three would be on the other side. They were responding to questions such as, "If you are or have a Jewish heritage, please cross to the other side." Or "If you were adopted, please cross to the other side."

"If you cannot be legally married to the person you love, please cross to the other side."

"If you ever felt prejudice because you are Black, Hispanic, Asian, please cross to the other side."

Some questions brought tears as people remembered hurts from years past. Some questions brought a silence that defied being broken.

The list of questions was endless. I found my feet moving in response to the questions even before I took the time to weigh in my mind whether or not I really wanted to answer them. I crossed that line again and again, acknowledging those parts of me that few people would ever know, at least no one from my professional life.

The final question was asked: "Were you ever a child?"

The entire group responded, palpably lightening up, as they confidently strode as a single body across the open area, reaching the red ribbon line on the opposite side. Laughter volleyed from one end of the line to the other. "We have all been children," they tossed the words and phrases from one to another. "This is an easy one to answer," they joked.

The pleasant noise of their voices followed their steps...at least until they turned around and saw me standing midway, only a few feet from the original starting place.

They all fell silent. Some gasped.

I was never a child. I did not possess a single memory from childhood that wasn't clouded by responsibility or fear. Yes, of course I lived through the years technically deemed the stages of childhood, but on this day, for this exercise, I could not honestly cross over to the other side.

It would have been easier if I had taken those steps, easier if I had pretended, as I always had, that my past was like everyone else's.

The exercise ended and I was enraged. During the mandatory debriefing with my buddy, Emilee, I voiced my absolute disgust with the exercise. "What possible good is it to dredge up all those old memories? Did I really need anyone to know about those times...sad times?"

"What happened?" she asked.

I struggled with my answer. It wasn't easy to explain, but she was my buddy and her concern was genuine. My voice was flat when I spoke. "My father left when I was ten. My parents had fought for years. Then he was gone in the middle of the night, leaving Mama with four kids, the youngest only nine months old. Uneducated, Mama hadn't worked for a living in years; she didn't have a chance in life. For years after that we lived with one relative or another. We lived in fear of doing something wrong, never feeling safe, never having a home of our own. I watched Mama lose her mind."

I was about to share more, then the rage returned. "I can't believe I didn't just lie, I can't believe I didn't walk over to the other side," I spat, as annoyed with myself as with the exercise. "It was all so stupid! I can't believe I let this stupid exercise get to me!"

Later, when we joined the sounding board of eight folks, my outrage pierced through the previously safe space we had all worked so hard to create. I had spent a lifetime tamping down and pushing away those horribly vulnerable, incredibly hurtful places from my past. To even acknowledge their existence felt like ripping off scabs from tender, never able to heal wounds.

"Why the hell do I need to be reminded of those times? Why now? Forty, fifty years later, after a lifetime of getting through them, ignoring them, denying they had any power over me?" I demanded, incredulous with the audacity of the prying.

My body shook. I fought back acid hot tears, felt them clog my throat and cut off my voice. I had never been so angry. My buddies tried to console me but I was lost in those dark sad times, surprised at the way those memories were so easily resurrected from that muddy, rank place deep down in my being. It was a place that I had never intended to visit again.

There was no salve that could calm my inflammation, no words that could appease me. Their worry was genuine but my pain remained, raw and unmanageable. I walked away from the group. They let me be alone.

Only I wasn't alone. Scenes from the past flooded my mind. Each time I had crossed that line to the other side, I relived some segment of that time. Hiding food for the baby. Learning to 'leave' my body when it couldn't escape prying hands. Seeing Mama grow smaller as she whimpered apologies, saying she was sorry for being alive and taking up space. Standing at a bus stop with all our belongings piled around us, three terrified kids looking up at Mama, who stood weeping, holding a toddler on her hip and not having a quarter in her pocket.

The images crawled back into my skull and danced in front of my eyes. Questions invaded my mind. *How could he? How could they? There was no one to stand up for that little girl—or her mother—or her little sister.*

When the entire class of 26 convened, my anger turned icy cold. I watched myself withdraw. I promised myself that I would go through the motions for the remaining days, I'd continue to show up for the meals and work groups, participate with my public face firmly in place, but nothing would reopen my heart. I would not trust that again, to anyone.

Two days later, by the time we had hiked 400 feet straight up the mountain, I sure wasn't thinking about the past. The present demanded my total attention and the physical effort was grueling. I was determined to hold my own; I wouldn't let anyone see me vulnerable again.

I thought back to the day before, when we had completed the rock wall climbing exercise. *If I made it up that rock, I can make it over this mountain!* I said over and over to myself, but by the time we reached the first mile marker of the hike, I wasn't so positive.

The climb continued. The time started to drag.

"You good?" one classmate would ask another.

"I'm good," the other would affirm.

It was the standard response. Before long, the "I'm good" exchange was heard between folks up and down the trail. It was an answer assuring all was well, physically, mentally.

We stopped midday. The light lunch didn't have much appeal. We forced water. The fatigue was setting in and we had another three miles to go. One kind soul had carried hard candy in his backpack and walked among us, offering a choice of flavors and types.

The hike resumed and we covered a few hundred feet before reaching a ledge that looked out over the range. We stood there, drinking in the sights of the undisturbed majesty of the mountains, treed in shades of green. We listened to the sound of wind blowing through the aspen, a sound unique to those tall white fragile looking trees. Huge boulders stood along the crest, defined by time and weather that chiseled them into gold and red and grey monuments.

I looked out over the indescribable, feeling the chilly breeze whip around my bare neck. As I marveled at the incredible sacredness, I realized I could not make it any farther. My heart dropped, my shoulders slumped and all of my resolve was gone.

I turned around and fell into Karun. He stood directly behind me and I realized he'd been standing there for a while, watching me, waiting patiently.

"Ready to let me carry it?" he asked with a smile.

I nodded. Surrender wasn't easy. I sighed loudly as he removed the straps and lifted the weight from my back. I felt the muscles around my shoulders slowly release, loosening their rigid, tight position. I stood up straight for the first time since the hike began and marveled at the sense of lightness. For a moment, I wondered if this was what it would feel like if I could let go of some of the boulders of responsibility that I carried in my day-to-day life.

A call from the hike leaders announced that break time was over. The group reassembled with some groaning as they pulled on their backpacks, fell into place, forming a line as we began the next phase of the hike. This part would be the most difficult of the uphill climb. We were so close to reaching the highest altitude of the trip—our ultimate goal: the summit.

Without the extra burden of weight, because of the help of a classmate, I could make it. Tired beyond words, out of breath but breathless with joy, I reached the summit. Time stopped. It was surreal to stand at the top and look out over the panorama of beauty. I reveled in joy. We hugged. We cried. We had done it! I had done it!

Suddenly I wasn't worried about making it down the other side of the mountain. We had been told that it would be the steepest and most physically challenging part of the hike as we made our way to the base camp. There we would spend the night having our solo experience, alone under snippets of tarp, with only our thoughts and an endless sky of stars for company.

The entire trip up the mountain to the summit and down to camp was 4.38 miles long and gained 1,850 feet. It took nine hours and five minutes. The financial analyst in the group timed it.

Later I would tell anyone who would listen that the ALF experience had saved my life. It was true. My classmates became the bridge that kept me sane through those two crazy years at work. They held me up during those long months between the time we almost lost the building and the time that would mark our worst year ever.

Even though few would ever know the full story of the little girl, they didn't have to. For those precious moments in time, on a mountain very far away, their caring surrounded and comforted the woman who was never a child.

Their caring was so unexpected and so unconditional. Looking back, I can see it started long before the hike began, but I didn't fully understand until Karun's generous offer. That's when I learned that it was okay to be vulnerable, to let someone else help with the load. I didn't always have to be the person who had all the answers, not with this group. And I could still be a leader in spite of it all. I had reached many summits in my life, but few would mean as much as this one.

As I walked carefully down the steep slope to camp, loving hands held branches aside for me. The guys waited, offering a shoulder for me to hold onto as I navigated treacherous rocky areas. The ground was covered with leaves, the surface was slick. Carefully, I placed each foot into the prints of those just ahead of me. With each step I took, I knew someone was ahead of me and behind me, ready to reach out and steady me—willing to catch me if I slipped or fell.

Finally, we were on level ground. I was lost in thought when Karun appeared beside me. We walked together and approached the camp.

"You good?" Karun asked, his eyes twinkling in merriment.

"Yes. Thank you," I responded. I was tickled, my smile was huge. "I'm good."

Chapter 25
The Lost Navigator

The grinding noise of metal elevator doors opening announced the arrival of another mass of people. The bank of elevators was hidden on both sides of the floor just off the long, colorless hallway that offered entry to Houston Criminal Courts 250 through 267.

As I watched the growing crowd of folks, I grew more and more anxious. Then I saw her. I knew it was Lynn the moment her slight, small figure rounded the corner. The light behind her hid her face in a shadow, but the swing of her long, shiny black hair was unmistakable. My heart lurched. It was the first time I had laid eyes on her since the day we discovered she had stolen from The Rose.

In the 25 year history of The Rose, no single event had shaken me so, destroyed my faith in people so completely.

I could still hear the tremble in Bernice's voice when she first called me, her anger vibrated through the telephone lines. She said it was actually Dixie who had made the initial discovery, who put two and two together. If it hadn't been for Dixie's curiosity about why she had not been paid for an outpatient surgery, Lynn's scam might have continued for a long time.

"I have no idea why I looked at the back of that patient's chart," Dixie told me the next day, "I never do that. But there it was, copies of the check made out to the surgery center and to the anesthesiologist. I thought that was odd. This patient had been so excited about her family and friends holding fundraisers, barbecue lunches, and bake sales. I had told her I didn't want a dime for doing her excisional biopsy, so when I saw the checks from the foundation I thought it was odd that I had not gotten one. It didn't add up. That was when I came to your office, but you were out so I went to Bernice."

I was out that afternoon, on the hour-long trip to deliver Patrick to the airport. He was headed out of the country for another stint in Doha, Qatar. When Bernice called, I had just dropped him off, knowing that for the next 24 hours there would be no communication with him. In a way that was good, it would take almost that long for us to know much of anything, except that something was very wrong.

The patient had paid for the surgery, but so had a foundation. There was no reason for both payments. The only answer was that Lynn must have been taking money from the patient.

The next day, Bernice called Lynn to the office. She admitted to taking $3,000 in cash from the patient. She swore it was the only time she had done it, insisting it had never happened before and would never happen again.

As Bernice was going through the process of terminating her, Lynn kept saying she would bring the money back.

"That would be good," Bernice said, "but you must leave, now."

Brahana walked Lynn down the stairs to her first floor office and watched her clean out her desk. It was a quick task; her few personal items barely filled up a cardboard box. Brahana escorted her out of the building and watched her drive away.

On Friday, Lynn returned to Bernice's office with $3,000.

"She handed me this envelope. It had $3,000 in cash inside it!" Bernice explained. "Brahana was in the room with me and I counted it out. Then Lynn stood there and wouldn't leave. I think she honestly thought she could get her job back." Bernice was obviously mystified.

"Who knows where she got this much cash! I took it, gave her a receipt for it and told her she would have to leave, now. It was bizarre, Dorothy, the way she kept standing there." Bernice paused, rethinking the encounter, "I did ask her again if she had stolen from anyone else, and she said no."

When Bernice was finally able to reach the patient, she confirmed that she had given Lynn $3,000 in cash, which the woman thought was pretty odd at the time. She had asked Lynn why she couldn't put the bill on a credit card, especially since her family had held the fundraisers and the money was in the bank. Lynn's response was that only cash was allowed in these kinds of cases.

It turned out that Lynn had instructed her staff to transfer all the difficult cases to her. "Difficult" meant those cases where the uninsured women needed excisional biopsies. Those were the ones who needed special funding by foundations or, if the patient didn't meet the low-income criteria, she had to pay for it herself at the discounted fee we negotiated with the surgery center.

Usually the surgeons would do the cases pro-bono if they knew the patient didn't have any money. The surgery center offered a flat fee for use of the surgery and recovery rooms, but seldom did the anesthesiologists reduce their standard rates. Very few of our women could afford even the discounted fees. The woman Lynn had swindled was one of the lucky ones who had family and friends able to host fundraisers.

Lynn had worked for us for eight years. She was a patient navigator, responsible for walking women through the bewildering maze of testing and surgery and treatment. Almost from the beginning, she had been a shining star; the patients genuinely cared about her and it seemed like the feelings were mutual. The Rose had paid for her to become certified by the state as a community health worker, and before long she was promoted to supervisor. Lynn's ability to speak five Asian languages was incredibly valuable and her tracking of patient care was above reproach. When her son was diagnosed with a medical problem, we agreed to adjust her work schedule to accommodate his need for her to be home in the afternoons.

As always, hindsight provides twenty-twenty vision. While it may not have been common knowledge, a lot of us knew Lynn had been having financial problems. We had heard about her husband being laid off, but it wasn't until she asked us for a $2,000 loan that we had a clue about the scope of her debt. Bernice was flabbergasted. First, it was a heck of a lot of money, and second, Lynn said she needed the check cut that day. They were about to foreclose on her home, she tearfully pleaded with Bernice.

But our policies were clear. We turned her down. Only in the rarest cases do we provide an advance, usually for an emergency, and even then the amount cannot be more than the paid time off that the employee had already earned.

Once the theft was discovered, we learned that Lynn had asked a lot of employees for money, and even convinced one of the doctors of her plight. The reasons she gave ranged from her brother having colon cancer and needing help to the same brother financing a restaurant in California and losing everything. In the week after we fired Lynn, 87 different creditors called her office, leaving demanding messages on her voicemail.

Every thief is a good liar. I guess they have to be to do what they do to people. By the end of that Friday, we had uncovered enough information to believe there could be more than one incident. The mantra 'We should have known' haunted me day and night as the investigation unfolded.

In the weeks and months that followed, I walked between two worlds. Sometimes my feet were firmly planted in my day-to-day responsibilities, attending meetings with potential funders, doing a presentation at a workshop, signing off on expenses, or reviewing and approving grant proposals. But most of the time, I was flayed by total disbelief. With each passing day, another dimension of Lynn's theft and dishonesty was discovered.

With each new finding, a new sense of betrayal pierced through me. Some days, I would end up in the bathroom washing my face, as if I could wipe away the strain that deepened every line. The constant effort of trying to keep my emotions so tightly in check ripped my insides apart. Anger and hurt leaked out through the fragile places of my being. I became robotic, simply doing things by rote, one foot ahead of the other, one task after another.

Talking to our legal counsel had been our first step. Jim was his usual available self, brilliant, quirky, even bordering on eccentric. He methodically recorded each happening and we agreed to visit on Monday and go over everything. But I woke up on Saturday morning knowing I couldn't wait even another 48 hours. I emailed him and he agreed to meet.

"Jim, we have to prosecute," I said, walking into his office. Since the first inkling of the theft that had been the big question—whether or not to prosecute.

He waited.

"I don't care if this is $3,000 or $30,000, it has to be turned over to the police." Later, thinking back on that conversation, I shuddered at the accuracy of the amount I had snatched out of thin air. "We can't let this ever happen again. We have to do the right thing."

For the next two hours, Jim, in his usual lawyerly manner, took me through the realities. He told me that a $3,000 theft might not even be worthwhile for the DA to consider. That fact hadn't occurred to me, a theft was a theft. Then he explained the law concerning cases involving a theft from a non-profit (or the elderly), and how those charges are automatically increased to the next penalty level. A misdemeanor becomes a felony, and the amount involved determines the degree of the felony.

He also reminded me that it would be a matter of public record. Oddly enough, he never questioned if I was prepared for the bad press, nor did he express any concerns he personally held as a board member about the publicity that we both knew was coming.

In 25 years we had never had a theft, at least not one like this. We'd fielded the occasional incident when an employee attempted to carry home a printer or we suspected someone was raiding the coffee supply, but nothing like this. All of our financial controls were in place—that was why it was such an opportunist crime and all the more frustrating. On the rare occasions when our patients paid anything at all for external services, any money exchanged was between the patient and the surgery center. The Rose was never involved in that step.

But Lynn had managed to find a way around the controls and

convinced at least one patient to hand over cash. In my heart of hearts, I knew we would find others.

By the time I left Jim's office, I was convinced we had to prosecute. It had started to rain and there was no let up until well past Monday, when Myrleen, our board chair, convened an emergency meeting of the board at noon. During the meeting they listened as Bernice took them through, step by step, the discovery and actions to date. They agreed that we had to prosecute but wanted us to find a criminal lawyer who could take the case directly to the DA's office.

Nearly every member conveyed an incident within their own businesses involving a theft. Someone said, "Look, Dorothy, even in the banking business with around the clock armed security guards, there are still robberies." Bernice had been through employee thefts in her other jobs, she knew these things happened, and that's why companies have insurance and background checks and all the other safeguards in place.

But it was different for me. This was a Rose employee, a patient navigator! Lynn's theft was a violation of everything a true patient navigator stands for, integrity and caring and all the incredible good they create through their daily duties. It was a patient navigator's job to guide each woman into care, help her overcome barriers, be her liaison, and walk with her on this journey. Navigators are the primary contact and bridge to treatment for patients. They help when no one else can and they work from the heart.

I felt personally responsible. As I listened to the board's attempts to reassure me, I couldn't shake off the feeling that everything I believed in about the goodness of people was close to being lost forever.

The staff meeting was harder than the board meeting. Everyone knew Lynn had been fired, but no one outside of the inner circle knew why. I told them that even though Lynn hadn't stolen directly from The Rose, we would prosecute the case to the full extent of the law. I emphasized that we would never allow this type of flagrant violation to go unpunished and would do everything in our power to make sure she never did that to anyone ever again. By the time I finished, half the crowd was in tears.

At this point, we had called enough patients to know that there were more who had brought cash to Lynn for their surgeries. Cash that they could barely afford, cash found by begging from relatives or friends.

Over the course of months, Lynn had systematically stolen from our most vulnerable patients. The full impact of that statement made me seethe inside: Our most vulnerable patients. She took advantage of their fear, preyed upon their ignorance.

There was no recourse with our insurance company. They said it was a theft from individual patients, not The Rose itself, so the underwriter officially closed the case. We had no claim. There was no way to use donated money to reimburse the patients, there seemed to be nothing that we could do to make things 'right.'

My friend and astrologer, Caroline, asked me, "What do you want to see happen, Dorothy? What is the best case scenario in your mind?"

I wanted three things. I wanted all the money returned to the patients; I wanted The Rose to come out of this stronger than before and our reputation not to be damaged in any way; and I wanted Lynn to never be able to do this to anyone again.

But I thought hard about the details involved in that last want. Did I really want Lynn to be punished to the full extent of the law? Did I want her to be locked away for years from her family? She was a mother with two small children. Did I want revenge or did I want justice?

Our patients, women fearing for their lives, had been scammed out of their grocery money. Our organization's stellar reputation and future ability to serve was at risk. Could there be any justice? For them? Any of us? Much less all of us?

People speculated about why she had done it, but oddly enough I didn't care why. In my mind there was no reason that could excuse such deliberately deceitful actions.

When we connected with the DA's office, we were led to the special Financial Crimes Division and Kaylynn, the Assistant DA. We could not have asked for a more competent prosecutor or compassionate human being. After hearing our story, she was outraged at the crime, empathetic to the victims and their families, and totally savvy about how The Rose as a non-profit was dependent upon the public trust. We knew instantly that we had our champion.

"It was such an egregious crime," she repeated again and again, infuriated that anyone would dare steal money from poor women facing a diagnosis of cancer.

By the time the investigation ended, we found 28 women who had been duped. One by one, Lynn's patients were sending their receipts to us and more thefts were uncovered. Some of the receipts looked very formal, printed out on Rose stationary, but others were handwritten on a lined pre-printed receipt, the type of pads that were available at any Office Depot store. Some receipts indicated the amount received was $500, others $2,500. Some of the women had not kept a receipt at all.

We discovered that Lynn had met some of the patients after

hours to collect the money. Those trusting souls never suspected the real reason for her willingness to come back to work in the late evening. They were so glad that they would not have to miss work to bring the money in; they were having a hard enough time taking off for the actual surgery.

Her system was almost flawless. Once she knew the application for funding was approved by the foundation and a check was on the way, she contacted the patient explaining that she was able to arrange their surgery at a discounted rate but they needed to bring the entire amount in to her—in cash. If the patient hesitated, she would tell them that their date couldn't be held for very long, since so many others also needed the service. They had to hurry up and bring her the money to secure the date.

One by one, they did as they were told.

Amazingly, barely a week after her termination, while we were still reeling, she reached out and slapped us in the face again. It was on a Friday, I was at a conference when my cell phone began to vibrate. By the time I reached the hallway, I saw that four messages had been left. I read the text "Call Brahana. ASAP." My stomach turned over. I dialed.

"Dorothy, you won't believe what just happened!" Brahana's voice was edged with anger. "Lynn showed up at Dr. Garcia's office! She was there to meet a patient who was waiting to talk with the doctor. Lynn acted like nothing had happened!" Her words raced over each other.

Apparently Lynn had shown up in the doctor's office knowing that one of our patients had an appointment that day. She told the patient she was there to help with the appointment and then tried to extort MORE money from her, in cash, on the spot. Of course, we had already called the patient to tell her Lynn no longer worked for us. By the time the doctor's receptionist realized what was going on and went to get the office manager, Lynn was gone.

I stood there holding the phone, speechless and in shock. Lynn was still trying to steal from our patients!

It was the afternoon of Friday the 13th when the police arrived at Lynn's home, stopping her as she was getting into her car on the way to a job interview. They handcuffed her, which was their standard procedure, and took her to jail. At 9:05 that next morning she stood before the judge for the arraignment. It was all captured on the courthouse internal TV system available to reporters on the police beat. By Monday morning the story had hit the internet, and by Monday afternoon I was fielding my first calls from the media.

With cameras rolling, microphones pushed into my face, and

reporters asking the same inane questions, somehow I remained honest and open but firm. "I will not share anything that could jeopardize our case," I said repeatedly. "The situation has been turned over to the DA and The Rose is focused on what we do best: taking care of women."

The media I could handle, but our funders were a different story. As I looked over the list of thirty plus major funders, I pushed hard against the door of dread. I was holding the phone, waiting for the first call to go through, when I became aware that my left hand was firmly covering my midsection. My body was instinctively moving into its protective mode, my hand trying to hold back the ocean of pain that flowed through my stomach.

Some of the funders had seen the news of the theft on TV, some had not. With only one exception, they were kind, gracious. A few offered stories of their own of times when their companies or organizations had experienced a theft. I was profoundly touched by those who expressed their genuine concern for me personally. They understood what an affront the entire situation was to me.

Only one funder wanted to know the details and implied any future funding could be in jeopardy, and summoned me to a mandatory meeting with their chair.

"We work so hard for the money we raise," the chairperson started the interrogation. "We need your guarantee that this will never happen again."

"Then our meeting is over," I replied, amazed at the steady resolve in my voice. "No one can guarantee that a theft will never occur." Throughout the hour-long meeting, I refused to grovel. To each statement reminding me that "Our board works so hard to raise the money," I thanked her and affirmed that we at The Rose worked equally hard to make sure that their money was used wisely, reminding her of our flawless stewardship of funds and reiterating that no donations from funders were involved in this matter. I was beginning to wonder how many times I would have to say that before she heard me.

The truth was, there really weren't many new procedures we could implement that could top those already in place. We had careful checks and balances for every monetary process and every point of sale transaction. I remember Kaylynn assuring me, "There wasn't anything you could have done that would have caught this. Lynn thought about it a long time. That's why there was such a time gap in the first case and the next one. She tested the system and waited, then, convinced she wouldn't get caught, did it again until it spiraled out of control. Simply put: she got greedy and sloppy. I've seen it happen over and over. She found the one soft spot in the system, the patient—those women who were so trusting of her. That was the only spot you could not have anticipated no matter how many procedures were in place." Her voice was determined.

Even though Lynn didn't physically steal from The Rose itself, she stole something precious from me and the other employees, something that could never be replaced: our innocence, our trust.

The time between the day of her arrest and the day we received the call from the DA's office telling us the terms of the deal was the longest two weeks of my life. It was early in the morning, just after 6 a.m., when I read the email telling me that Kaylynn was close to reaching a deal with Lynn's attorney. Lynn had admitted to having a gambling problem.

Kaylynn said Lynn would immediately pay full restitution to The Rose for all patients. Apparently her husband was willing to cash out his 401(k) to pay her debts. Secondly, she would serve a probated sentence in which she spent at least six months in prison (on weekends, three days of credit at a time). And thirdly, Lynn would write individual letters of apology to the patients she stole money from. If she failed to meet the terms of the arrangement, then she would be subject to the full penalty under the law for her offense, which could be up to twenty years in prison.

As I reread the third condition, I realized I could not allow Lynn to have any contact with our patients for any reason. A letter of apology to them would be like salt thrown on a wound. I nixed that section but agreed to the rest.

The deal was struck, and on Friday, June 1, 2012, at 9 a.m. sharp, Bernice stood in front of a window inside the court house to pick up the cashiers' check for $37,098. She was downright giddy when she called me.

"It is in my hands." Her voice was eager and quick. "And will soon be in the bank! We can start issuing checks immediately to the patients!"

I had to smile at the lilt in her words. It was nice to smile again.

The greatest irony of all was that Lynn's attorney was someone who knew The Rose and our mission well. In fact, when she was a law student, uninsured and needing a mammogram, she had turned to us for help.

The day soon came for sentencing, and I sat on that hard metal bench, waiting for the courtroom to open. I watched Lynn leaning against the wall. Her eyes met mine, I looked for any indication of remorse but she quickly looked away. Inside the courtroom, Lynn sat three rows in front of me. Her case was announced and she approached the bench, her attorney stood beside her. I struggled to hear the proceedings.

The accusation was read, Lynn pled guilty and the judge announced the sentence: thirty days of city jail time, six years of probation, some community service, and monthly meetings with Gamblers Anonymous. The judge's voice grew louder, "And you are to write a letter of apology to your ex-employer." I could see the judge pointing a finger at Lynn, "Your ex-employer, who was kind enough to give you employment, which you repaid by stealing from them."

A lump rose in my throat, I forced back the tears and willed myself to a state of calmness.

A tall uniformed policeman took Lynn by the arm and guided her to a counter, where she signed something, then he continued to move her to an exit behind the gated section. She disappeared to the place where criminals go.

When all was said and done, only 45 days had passed from her arrest to the day she went to jail. One of my attorney friends said that everything that had happened to move this case forward was nothing less than a miracle. Seldom, if ever, is the money returned, much less the entire amount. Seldom does the justice system move so quickly. I nodded as she recounted each miracle, large and small.

Kaylynn bristled at the actual time Lynn would spend in jail, but she added that if Lynn broke parole, she would go to jail for a very long time.

One of our board members said, "There was no happy ending to this, only an ending."

He was correct.

Chapter 26
The Last Dream Was About Mama

It was August, 2012, when Mimi Swartz's article, "Mothers, Sisters, Daughters, Wives," appeared in the *Texas Monthly Magazine*. It was an account of the 2011 session of the state legislature that slashed family planning funds, passed the sonogram law, and created the sad state of affairs for women's health in Texas. Her article foreshadowed events that convinced my friends on the East Coast that Texas really was a third world country, at least when it came to attitudes about women and how laws that impacted them were decided. Mimi's article predicted a bleak time ahead and the possibilities haunted me.

"The last dream was about Mama," I said to Patrick, warming my hands around a cup of hot coffee. "She had died and her body was in a recliner and I was trying to make funeral arrangements when her eyes opened."

Recounting my nightly dreams to my husband was our morning ritual. He'd attempt an interpretation and we'd discuss them. That night I had had six dreams. "This dream was somehow connected to the other one about you and I living in a rental house. It was plain and simple. We had lost our beautiful home and were in this house and couldn't get to our money or valuables," I said.

"What does a house mean in a dream?" he asked. "It isn't energy, is it? That's a car."

"A house means the self, the essence of someone," I responded automatically. "I think I know what prompted that dream. It was an old tape playing in my head yesterday when we were talking about your work."

Patrick was trying to decide whether to continue working overseas for a group that kept him hanging until the last moment before confirming when his next stint would commence. It had been a long four years of his back and forth sojourns, never knowing if he would be over there a month or six months or at all. The last two trips had ended abruptly with unplanned schedule changes, and he was in limbo waiting to see if he would be returning.

"Old tapes?" he asked.

"Yes. Yesterday, when we were talking about your job and what would happen if you didn't go back overseas, that it could mean no work, and to me 'no work' means 'no house.' But even when the thought raced through my mind, I realized it was old stuff. From nine or ten years."

"More than nine or ten years ago," he said, looking confused. "We've been together nearly twelve years, Darling." He smiled at his statement but his eyes were still questioning.

"No, I meant when I was nine or ten years old. That was when Daddy had his first heart attack and couldn't work full time. That was when we lost the house, the one they were buying in the Heights. It was a really nice house—at least nice for middle class folks. I had my own room, with all my pretty furniture, the blond dresser with the round mirror," my voice sounded small. "But he got sick and they had to leave—I'm sure it went into foreclosure, some company bought it and tore it down.

"We moved to a rental house, a tiny, dirty place at the end of a road that was out in the sticks, in the middle of nowhere over on 34th street. That's when Mavis was born. Mama must have been miserable. The rental house only had four rooms, five with the bathroom. We lived there about ten months before Daddy got really sick, lost his job and left. I was ten."

I fought back the other memories of that time after Daddy left. Days of watching Mama cry and pace the floor. She never did learn to drive, so the car just sat there. I was the oldest and kept wondering what we would do when the food ran out. We didn't have any neighbors close by. It was two long weeks before Mama called her sister and asked for help. I think she always thought Daddy would come back. It was another week before her sister came, sold what she could, loaded up a truck with what little belongings we had left—my pretty dresser was long gone—and took us, four unruly, screaming kids and a woman numb from crying, to the Texas Panhandle.

"No work, no house…no home," I said, looking over at Patrick, "an old tape," I smiled.

"In the dream about Mama," I went on, "she was dead and lying on the recliner when her eyes opened up and then she started moving around. Her body was real thin, like Mama was when she died, all skin and bones. She got up and sort of jerked around as she tried to walk. I went off to find someone to help and when I returned she was gone. So the search began for her. Every time I found her, she would be dead again, but then she would not stay dead and would be gone again. Somewhere in the dream there was a guy eating a big steak dinner, it was on a plate at the table where she sat, only she couldn't have any of it. She was dead."

Patrick stared at me, shaking his head. "So, Mama won't stay dead?" he questioned.

"I don't know if that's what it means." I stopped as a memory from the past rushed in. "Actually, the steak is the real clue. Somehow this dream is connected to that article about women's healthcare in *Texas Monthly Magazine*, the one Mimi Swartz wrote."

He nodded, he had also read it.

I was still struggling with my response to that article. First I felt enraged, then frustrated, then sad. Mimi's article left no doubt that women's healthcare was on the bottom rung of importance as far as our state legislature was concerned. Every time I thought about the harsh reality of the total insanity of the system in Texas, I shuddered. There was an almost certain knowing in my soul that it won't change, can't change.

On that morning with Patrick, I continued, "I remember the only time as a kid when I actually understood how truly poor we were. Oh, there had been a few other times, but nothing major. I lived in my own world with my books. I knew we didn't dress like the other kids, we didn't have a daddy around, and nobody else's mother had to use a taxi for a monthly trip to the grocery store. But for the most part I didn't really know just how poor we were until the time we went to see Uncle Buddy and Aunt Ernestine at their farm in Franklin, twenty miles or so out of Hearne. Do you remember the time we went through that area?"

Patrick nodded.

"Anyway, we were at their home and it was so pretty, everything was in its place. Their primary home was in a small town in East Texas. Uncle Buddy had done well in his life; folks said everything he touched turned to gold. He always wore his Stetson ten gallon hat." I glanced at Patrick. "He looked a lot like the state representative in that picture, the one of the bill being signed into law, from Mimi's article. He was the one wearing the big cowboy hat."

Returning to that time long ago, I said, "I remember there was a bowl of green grapes sitting on the counter. Grapes were my favorite but we never had them at our house; that was a luxury. So I waited, hoping they would be offered to us. Of course, my sister Joyce, always the bold one among us, just reached over and took a handful. Mama scolded her, my aunt put them in the refrigerator and none of us got any of them." I half smiled.

"It was Uncle Buddy who had reopened the old family home in Hearne, Grandpa's house, so we would have a place to live. Mama and four kids, we lived on Grandpa's retirement and whatever extra Uncle Buddy put into the pot. Looking back, I realize that arrangement was probably a good trade off. Grandpa had a built in caregiver. He didn't have to stay with his grown children anymore and they didn't have the cost of putting him in a nursing home. Anyway, that's how we had a place to live for three years—until Grandpa died."

On that day, at my aunt and uncle's country home, Uncle Buddy was sitting on this oversized leather couch and chewing on a big cigar, talking to Mama. I can still recall his exact words. "Well, Sister, when I have a big ol' juicy steak, I don't want anything put on it. No steak sauce. Stuff like that spoils the taste of the meat. I like my steak thick and cooked rare." He sucked on the cigar, blew out a big blue stream of smoke and looked up, watching it drift to the ceiling. He smiled.

I remember staring at him and thinking, *My Mama hasn't had a steak for as long as I can remember. How could he be talking about something like that?* We lived on macaroni goulash, beans, and cornbread, and had meat maybe once a week on Sunday after church. A small roasted chicken that somehow Mama made go round for six people—once a week if the money lasted—was the highlight of our week, and this man is talking about eating steak?

Pure rage engulfed my little body. But rage gave way to tears that filled my eyes as I watched Mama. She never missed a beat or let on to him that, for her, steak was a distant memory. Her hands smoothed her simple cotton dress. She looked up at him and, with a huge smile, agreed, "You're right, Buddy, there isn't anything that needs to be put on a good piece of beef!"

I was the only one who had seen her hands tremble. I knew that forced laugh of hers well. Something made her glance over at me and the shock on my face must have alarmed her. Her eyes bored through me, vivid blue eyes intense with their message—'Don't you dare say a thing.'

I couldn't believe his insensitivity. Like the pioneer men described in the *Texas Monthly* article, as far as he was concerned he'd taken care of his sister and he'd done the right thing by her. Too bad she didn't have steak to eat now and then, but in reality that part of her world would never have occurred to him. Not what she ate, or how she managed to care for four kids, or if she was ill, especially the last one. She had 'woman's problems,' the family would whisper later. "No one else in the family ever had that. Must be something wrong with her," they repeated knowingly to each other.

Mama died way too young. She was uninsured, poor, didn't have a doctor or a place to go. The bleeding, long after monthly bleeding had stopped in her life, was the clue that something was wrong, deadly wrong. The bleeding she ignored, the pain she couldn't. She was embarrassed to go to a poor person's clinic, embarrassed to have to tell someone about the bleeding.

On the day she finally went to the doctor, she made sure she douched so there wouldn't be any odor. There was an odor all right, but nothing a douche could erase. The cancer had already spread, and with it came an unmistakable smell.

She was out of her mind with worry. Of course, her number one worry was the last child still at home, depending on her meager earnings as a housekeeper.

But by the time she had exploratory surgery, the cancer had raged through her body, ravaging every possible living organ, sucking out life as easily as those men in their ten gallon hats suck at their cigars. The doctor closed her up and sent her home.

There wasn't a system in place to be sure she could have a pap smear. The test existed but Mama never had one. Had a system for care been available, it could have meant finding her cervical cancer earlier, and undoubtedly, it would have saved her life.

That was 42 years ago.

If she were alive today, her fate would be the same. After all, the Uncle Buds of the state are determining what is 'good' for her and her health.

She spent the last weeks of her life in a charity hospital. I was with her, leaning in close to her face, hearing her hoarse whispers asking about the kids and assuring her they would be all right.

Those last three days were filled with listening to each exhale become more ragged, each inhale spaced further apart. Three days of watching her gaunt face contort when the nurses tried to move her skinny boney body racked with pain. Three days of staring into those steel blue eyes, filled with terror, silently begging me to help her leave.

Mama's dead, but she dies again and again—as does a part of every woman—with the passage of another legislative bill that eliminates a civil right, with each decision to close or 'adjust down' another service for women's health. Each day when a woman is not valued as a human being, Mama dies again.

Chapter 27
Rejections and Pink Anger

It wasn't the rejection, but it was.

It wasn't how much we had counted on this particular grant, but it was.

It wasn't the hope we had when the foundation had said that waiting until their January meeting would give our request a much better chance of being funded, but it was.

It was one more denial in a stream of denials that would worry anyone in non-profit work.

Someone once said The Rose just wasn't "glamorous" enough to draw down the big bucks. Maybe it's true. After all, what was glamorous about being the messenger?

Treatment, now that was a different story. Being a treatment center meant lots of funding, especially for buildings and research. Helping someone go from illness to health was different.

Telling someone that she had a terminal disease simply was not endearing. Yet, every year we told over 350 women that their life was about to change forever. We told them the biopsy was conclusive—the medical term used is "positive for cancer." What a strange mixture of words: positive and cancer in the same phrase. And every year, nearly two-thirds of those 350 women faced this diagnosis knowing they did not have medical insurance. Their recovery depended not only on the stage of their disease, but also on them qualifying for the state program that provided treatment.

The old adage that surviving cancer depended on how good one's insurance was and the amount of money in one's bank account was never truer than in the fall of 2012.

So when Trina said the foundation had turned us down, I literally doubled over, catching my midsection with one hand. For days, the pain from that imaginary blow lingered, bringing with it very physical symptoms, nausea and stomach upset. That evening, long after my daily sharing of events with Patrick, we sat side by side on the couch and a huge sob caught in the back of my throat. He looked at me. I shook my head. *How silly of me,* I thought. *I've been through grant denials before. This one is no worse than any others over the last 26 years,* I argued with myself, yet somehow it was.

This funding could have launched us on our way to Solid Ground, the tagline of our fundraising campaign. I remembered how attentively the foundation's trustees had listened to our presentation. The understated yet obvious wealth in that room bounced throughout the exquisitely appointed meeting area and its equally well-clad members. Having an audience with the trustees was a good sign. We met their criteria, they said.

It was odd that they didn't seem excited about the sustainability part of our proposal. Our prospectus showed how an increase in the number of insured women, reaching the ultimate ratio of three insured to one uninsured, would nearly cover program costs. Those costs were no small change; providing a full range of screening, diagnostic, and navigation services to over 9,000 uninsured women meant raising over $2.5 million each year.

How many times had we been told that we needed to be more sustainable? That message had been voiced by this group often enough, especially when they told us not to think of them as an annuity, something that could be sought year after year.

But obviously, it didn't matter in the end.

Over the past two years, I had watched Trina struggle against the rejections, second guessing her work and approach. It never seemed like she fully celebrated the approvals and she certainly had her fair share of them, her work was in the 58% approval range. For a grant writer, that's darn good. But these days, she never took time to stop and enjoy her successes because she was mentally too far along in creating the next proposal and juggling work priorities against looming 'hard' deadlines.

Trina was a novelty among grant writers. In her past life, she had been a development director for a large foundation and she had plenty of experience in all aspects of fundraising. She loved this job, she assured me often, but I wondered how she kept any sense of sanity. I knew what she was going through. I had been the grant writer for The Rose for most of its existence and was well aware of how rejections wore down one's confidence.

Writing of any kind requires space. Grant writing requires a Sherlock Holmes mindset for deciphering funders' goals, missions, and specific allowances, both written and implied. The greatest challenge was determining how the grantor's 'stated priority' aligned with the grantee's goals and requests. One funder might list "Issues of women and children" as a priority concern, while eliminating funds for health issues of that same population. Another may only fund capital equipment in the third round of their annual process, but fail to be specific about the dates of their meetings.

Some do not accept unsolicited proposals and require that the grantee be "among the preselected list." How to get on that list remains a mystery. So grant writers venture forth, submitting a letter asking to be considered for consideration to the list. It gets tricky. Many times the request for consideration receives a flat out rejection or no response at all—either way, it's a bust and drives the grant writer further down crazy lane.

This rejection marked the second large request to be turned down that year. A third proposal, requesting an equally large amount, sat pending with another group. But their grant officer had already warned us that she could not recommend the entire amount.

The next day, Trina and I strategized other possibilities. I watched her turn the sheets of paper in each folder. A beautiful woman with shoulder length dark hair, Trina was utterly organized and methodical in the way she gathered and presented information. Her professional approach to work didn't quite match her personality. She could carry an outrageously cute purse or wear a black and lavender spider-shaped hat to celebrate Halloween as easily as she could don a suit and talk to a funder. She could boot scoot better than most to a Country Western song, was always ready to volunteer for karaoke, and was the first person to try to teach me how to twerk.

But today, she was all tight lipped, her elbows pointed out from her stiff body at awkward angles as she clenched the folders tightly in her crossed arms.

She asked, "What are we going to do?"

I tried to smile. "We'll figure something out."

As my mind raced through different scenarios, I struggled with the lack of possibilities.

Within the next two months, we would hear bad news from Susan G. Komen-Houston, but every grantee on their list had been forewarned. The national PR fiasco had resulted in a loss of supporters, and in Houston it meant they would not reach their goals and therefore their grantees would not receive full funding.

At the same time, our number one funder, the Cancer Prevention Research Institute of Texas, known as CPRIT, was embroiled in what had turned into a huge legal issue following an audit that revealed possible misappropriation of funds. The rumors were running rampant—no new grants were being awarded and previous grants were totally dependent upon the legislature allocating funds.

The Rose was one of the first organizations to receive a CPRIT grant; it gave us the ability to serve 2,300 more women that first year. Three years later, CPRIT funding would mean serving 6,000 women from 24 counties in Southeast Texas.

No one had a cure for cancer yet. The best we could do was find it early and move those women quickly into the right treatment. Early detection, timely treatment, accessible care, it all added up to survival.

If the rumors about CPRIT had even a smidgen of truth, none of those 6,000 women would receive care, not even the most basic screening. Their lives depended on the people who had nothing to lose but a vote.

Two large requests had been denied by previous supporters, another equally large one postponed until June. Komen was sure to reduce funding, and who knew if CPRIT would continue or not. Each event created another floor in this Tower of Babel going on in my mind. But unlike the biblical tower, this one wasn't headed heavenward; it was tottering badly, swaying between the realities, lives lost to no funding.

After a long sleepless night, I dragged into work the next day, exhausted. I'm sure other CEOs would read these words and laugh. After all, a couple of rejections aren't the end of the world. I pushed away from my desk, announcing to myself that it was time for a walkabout.

Seeing patients in the waiting area always reminded me of our mission, and on many occasions someone would call out to me. I loved seeing one of our loyal patients. We'd share old memories, places and people—"I had my first mammogram in that tiny storefront office," they would say, or "Do you know Regina has done my mammogram for eight years now?" Their pride at being part of our history was contagious and uplifting. But today the atmosphere in the overcrowded reception area was tense and there wasn't a familiar face among them.

My next stop was the doctors' reading area. I could usually count on Dr. Parsons to have discovered something new in the regulations that he didn't like or some new equipment that he did like and we needed to buy. Today he was on a tirade about an old issue with our patient tracking system and I simply didn't have the patience to listen. I quickly made my exit.

Dixie stopped me to tell me her latest success story in weight management, noting that if only Dr. P would stay away from the candy he could lose weight and get a handle on his diabetes. "I forbade anyone to bring him any more treats," she harrumphed. Then she continued with, "You do realize that he and I are the same age and he never feels as good as I do. He says I must have good genes. Ha! I told him I get up every morning at 4 a.m. to do my exercises and I keep my weight down." Her eyes squinted and she asked, "Don't you think that has something to do with it?"

I nodded, and gave thanks as I heard her being paged to go to the ultrasound area.

Tiring. It was all so tiring. Dr. P and his chronic complaining, Dixie and her one woman battle against the bulge, hers and everyone else's. Me and my never-ending search for funding. It was all tiring. We had become tiring. What happened to the days of dreaming and possibilities?

I shuffled down the hall and into the imaging area, nodding to the techs as they guided their patients in or out of the mammogram suites. It was good to see their smiles.

Next, I roamed through the back offices and waved at the schedulers. Maribel called out to me to stop. I had barely stepped into her office when she asked, "What's up? You look down."

So much for my fake smile.

Maribel had only been with us for a year, and for the entire time we had struggled with a schedule that was booked out for four to five weeks for diagnostic appointments such as ultrasounds and mammograms that require a physician to be present. She once told me, "There are some days when it gets pretty hard to take, the patients are so upset when I tell them they have to wait. We schedulers are the ones they yell at."

I knew the constant tension was wearing our staff down. It was another example of our need for more capacity. A new ultrasound system cost nearly $200,000; a new mammogram machine was close to $500,000. The truth was, we could install ten new machines, but without more physicians they would all be useless.

Even if we could find physicians who were willing to do mammography only, they wanted a multi-year guarantee, somewhere between $350,000 and $400,000 a year with eight weeks paid vacation. I didn't share that part of our problem with Maribel or tell her that our biggest challenge with bringing on another physician was convincing our other docs of the need—they saw competition instead of added capacity. Without funds to expand capacity, we would never catch up, and if we spent what little reserve we had, we could be cash poor within months. All those thoughts raced through my mind before I could answer her question.

"Oh, we just had another rejection…from a funder."

"Rejection. I don't like that word," she frowned.

"Neither do I," I smiled.

"Other grants will come in," she said as I turned to move on. Then she called out after me, "Just remember, we are in the business of saving lives!"

In the months ahead, we would receive more rejections than ever before. In the end, we had to face facts. Ours was a 'disease specific' organization, and in the funding world the focus had moved to primary care and Federally Qualified Health Centers.

Part of the drop in our funding was because funders were convinced (or so they said) that the Affordable Care Act would result in everyone having insurance. There would no longer be a need to support non-profits providing healthcare to the uninsured. Some foundations were waiting or applying their resources to more global issues, homelessness or hunger or environmental causes. "After all," the head of a local major company had said in private, "those homeless people on the streets aren't good for attracting new businesses to Houston."

The truth was, the only way for the Marketplace Healthcare Exchange to be successful was if each state passed and funded Medicaid Expansion to offset care to the poorest. Texas didn't expand.

People falling below the 138% poverty level were supposed to be able to use their state's expanded Medicaid plan. Nearly half of the 22,000 uninsured women we served in the past three years were in that category, which meant they still didn't have insurance. The other half fell between the 138 and 200% poverty level. That group was supposed to purchase some type of coverage or face a fine.

The uninsured aren't going away. It could be years before the Affordable Care Act makes a real change for them. Trying to simplify the most convoluted and complex health reform to ever be implemented in our nation is difficult.

The other reason for the drop in funding was the fallout from Pink Anger. A grants officer at one national breast cancer foundation said, "I had hoped this year would be better but people are still angry at pink. We're down another 20% in fundraising. Everyone in the breast cancer world has suffered. I know of two groups that had to close completely." His words took some of the sting out of hearing that our $250,000 request had been denied, but not much. They had been a major supporter for nearly a decade.

I was tired of The Rose being punished because of the "angry at pink" sentiment that permeated many segments. It was the result of Komen's decision to not fund Planned Parenthood. The public outcry had been huge.

Trying to decipher the Komen fiasco wasn't easy. People ask me: Was it political? Poor judgment? My response: Who knows?

The situation had dragged on for months and I cringed whenever I received another rejection stating, "Our foundation has refocused its attention on more broad needs of the community and will no longer fund disease specific organizations." Read: "breast cancer."

One denial came from a 23-year funder, someone who had stuck by us through thick and thin. Even though their mission was women and poverty, now they were "refocusing" their funding strategy. I don't doubt they had a new strategy, but since their executive director had told me that she would never participate in a Komen Walk again, it didn't take being a rocket scientist to read between the lines on that one.

People were angry about Komen's decision, but ironically those same people didn't necessarily turn around and fund Planned Parenthood.

I heard way too many people say Komen didn't care anymore. I thought back on all the years that Komen had been our top funding partner and a part of every step of our growth. There were thousands of women they had funded for screening or diagnostics or treatment. They understood that need. Not care? Doubtful.

I knew the people at the local affiliate, I had lunch with them, had been to their baby showers, walked beside their volunteers, like Ann, for over two decades at the Race for a Cure. Ann had been a charter member of our support group, The Rosebuds, helping us start it in 1993. She represented the best in Komen volunteers, women like Heather and Ginny the best in Komen staff. No, I was certain that those people cared. I'd bank my life on it and I had, over the years, banked a lot of other women's lives on their caring.

But the timing of the whole thing was curious. The story goes that Komen had made the decision about not funding Planned Parenthood in late September, to be effective the first of the year. That decision didn't make the 6 o'clock news, but in a way that made sense. October is National Breast Health Month. Komen owns that month with all the pink ribbon events. Planned Parenthood would have been crazy to protest Komen's decision during that month.

After October, any announcements competing with the Holiday noise would have been lost to the public. Move forward to the end of January, the slowest, dullest time of the year, and suddenly the media was full of stories about Komen slashing funding to Planned Parenthood. Komen was obviously caught unaware. Their affiliates throughout the nation were learning more from the media than their headquarters, while Planned Parenthood clinic staff were well informed and their leaders were well prepared with their message.

To an outsider looking in, it was a communications nightmare and nothing Komen did in response quelled the swell of anger towards them. Even though Komen reversed their decision and returned to funding Planned Parenthood, the damage was done.

The sad thing is that not one of the Planned Parenthoods in the Houston area had ever applied to Komen for funding. Planned Parenthood had always sent women to The Rose for their mammograms. Komen had been our largest funder for two decades and Planned Parenthood was a resource for our women who didn't have physicians, those women needing referrals.

Believe me, there were just as many people upset at Komen for reversing their decision as there were who were mad when they first eliminated funding. I've heard it both ways. Just as I've heard folks saying, "Yes, Komen messed up, but it's time to move on."

In Houston, the funding gained by Planned Parenthood amounted to covering about 50 mammograms compared to the 2,500 Komen would normally fund at The Rose and another 1,500 they funded for other agencies. The fallout ensured that the Houston affiliate wouldn't meet their fundraising goals and would have to cut funding. So in my book, the ones who really suffered were the women we wouldn't serve.

That year, and every year since, awards from Komen and other foundations continued to decrease. Each year, we search for replacement funding—not likely as long as this anger against pink is fueled.

Each year, we must tell more women that we don't have enough funding to cover their annual mammogram, the same women we worked so hard to educate in the first place and who put away their fears and embarrassment about asking for help and starting screening. The same women who will receive an annual reminder letter (that we are required to send), only to learn we can't help them.

So I ask again, "In the end, who wins and who loses?"

Chapter 28
Capitol Beat

The Texas Capitol building in Austin is a towering mass of huge reddish limestone blocks. From its multiple rows of wide stone steps to the top of its cupola, it is a building fraught with antiquity and presence. Huge lush sections of green grass and giant oak trees with limbs that reach far over the web of private inner circle streets create the perfect frame for the state's seat of power.

On a wet drizzly day in March of 2013, I pushed through the massive fifteen foot tall wooden doors and took my place in a long snaking line of people, all waiting to be searched for dangerous articles. Looking past the security area with its hooded x-ray scanners and conveyor belts, I was struck by the enormity of the corridor that weaved through the first floor to the rotunda.

Polished pecan colored wood graced the walls, office doors, and rows of benches that lined the walls. Two Texas Rangers, their stance stiffer than their freshly starched khaki uniforms, wore cowboy boots and hats. They stared into the crowd. Holstered guns that hugged their thighs promised law and order would be maintained. It was the frontier, the Capitol, an ever-changing political landscape that often devoured the well-meaning and hid the wicked. It was a fickle place, loyal to no one, and those who managed to stay in office sported superhuman endurance, thick skin, and a closet filled with favors owed.

It was the second month in a row for me inside this building. In February, I had testified before both the House Finance and Appropriations subcommittee and the Senate committee on behalf of CPRIT, stressing the need for it to continue.

It was easy to size up which representatives and senators were against reissuing the bonds that would fully fund the program. After all, $300 million was a lot of money, and many other hungry coffers could be filled with it. But the voters had approved the use of those funds specifically for the purpose of finding a cure for cancer and there really wasn't a way to reallocate the funds without facing a huge public outcry.

No one wanted to fight that battle. But they could drag out the final decisions until the end of the legislative session, which was four long months away. Or they could decide to sit out a session, making no decisions as the problems were "studied."

The Texas legislature met biannually for 180 days, from January through May, and they considered thousands of bills. Doing nothing until they went in session again in 2015 would eliminate CPRIT funding for two years and essentially kill most programs.

Testifying to the House committee was nerve racking enough, but it paled in comparison to sitting before Senator Jane Nelson and eight other senators. The Senate Chamber was exceedingly more elegant than the House Appropriations Meeting Room and the power that room contained made it even more impressive. Senator Nelson's Bill 192 would revamp CPRIT and hopefully save it before the session was over.

I only had two minutes to present my testimony and I dove in with, "If there is any doubt about the importance of CPRIT, let me show you." I stood up and whipped out a two by two foot map showing our part of Southeast Texas and the 24 counties that The Rose served.

Setting the poster on the edge of the table, I pointed to the middle of the map. "These seven counties, the ones colored in light pink, represent the service area we covered before CPRIT funding. Let me assure you that there is no lack of uninsured in Harris County," I pointed at the map, "but the real need is in the rural communities. The areas in the deeper pink color," my hand now moved down the side of the poster closest to me, "are the counties that we were able to serve with the first CPRIT funding—that meant 2,300 women were screened and, when needed, had diagnostic services."

Next I directed their attention to the opposite side of the poster, "And these counties in the darkest pink are the ones added from the most recent CPRIT grant—which will mean another 6,000 women served in the three year period."

One of the senators boasted, "Nine of those counties are in my district."

"Then you are well aware, Senator, of the real need in these counties," I said.

He nodded.

I continued, "There is no way a small organization like The Rose could possibly serve so many women without CPRIT funding. Mobile mammography is how we do it, and there isn't another group that could reach these areas. Believe me, when we go into a rural area, our days are always packed and we don't have no-shows. The women are so glad to have the services."

I closed by saying, "We diagnosed breast cancer in 68 women during our first two years, but more importantly 29 of them were from a first time mammogram. Twenty one were in women under fifty years old, all of them have children." I paused, looking at each senator. "It hurts my heart to think that even one dollar of CPRIT funding wasn't used correctly," another short pause, "but on behalf of these women and the thousands we have yet to serve, thank you for caring about the women of Texas and for keeping CPRIT alive and strong." I glanced at the timer on the table. I'd done it! My testimony was under two minutes.

Fast forward to March.

The Breast Health Collaborative of Texas was hosting its first Advocacy Day. Forty members from all over the state, many at their own expense, had traveled to Austin. They were a mixed group that included certified community health workers, coordinators of Breast and Cervical Cancer Services (BCCS) programs, health educators, and at least ten breast cancer survivors. They came from East Texas, the Rio Grande, Houston, Austin, and the Panhandle. Only a handful had ever been to the Capitol before.

I was proud of the Collaborative. The Rose had been a big part of birthing it. Our tag line said it all: "So no woman diagnosed with breast cancer ever goes untreated." I had collected a few key players, found about $10,000 in funding, and we held the first Breast Health Summit in 2005. Throughout those early years of growing the Collaborative, The Rose provided the space and resources, and I wrote the grants to support it.

By 2013, the Collaborative had earned its own non-profit status and had its own executive director. It had moved its offices out of The Rose and grown its membership to over 400.

On the night before our Advocacy Day, our communications person, Karen, led the group through training and shared some tips about visiting Capitol offices and appropriate etiquette.

"Just because an aide looks like she or he is twelve years old, don't blow them off. They carry a lot of weight with the legislators. And they may be the only chance you have to get your message heard. Remember, it's your story they will remember, not your name or who you represent." She paused, looked down at a young woman sitting in the front row, stuck out her hand, and said, "The very first breast cancer survivor I ever interviewed was a young woman about your age. She was 21 and had a one-year-old baby. Hers was a tough cancer but

I'm glad to tell you that she's alive today because of The Rose and the state's funding for the Breast and Cervical Cancer program. Hi, I'm Karen Campbell and I work for The Rose, and I'm here to ask for the senator's support of BCCS."

Karen looked out at her stunned audience, and said, "There, THAT'S how you get your story out first."

Next up, we presented priority issues, the funding of CPRIT and BCCS and introducing reimbursement for community health workers.

"Be careful," I warned, "don't associate the BCCS program with Medicaid or someone will start opposing it." That message might have sounded crazy, but after all, this was Texas. There was still a law on the books forbidding women from owning a vibrator. It had been there since the late 1800s. My warning about BCCS was needed. I sure didn't want anyone opening debate about it being just another form of Medicaid that needed to be eliminated. BCCS was the only program that included treatment services for women.

"Can you imagine being diagnosed with breast cancer and there not being a single program in Texas that could help? Before we had the BCCS treatment arm, we had to beg physicians and hospitals for surgeries, chemotherapy, and radiation treatments." I was preaching to the choir, but the questions from them afterwards confirmed most did not realize the full implications or limitations of the programs.

Next, we covered obtaining reimbursement for community health workers. Everyone in that room knew that CHWs, or patient navigators, are near and dear to my heart. I looked out at the sea of faces. "CHWs keep people out of the emergency rooms and help them find health homes. Access to care is more of an issue than ever before. Reimbursement is the key! It simply HAS to happen!" I paused, a little embarrassed by the level of my booming voice. I took a deep breath and ended with, "I firmly believe that CHWs are the future of healthcare in this country! That's what you are asking for—the future!"

The history of patient navigators is similar to social workers. There was a time when social workers were volunteers, helping people find resources; then social workers had to be certified to be able to work, just like CHWs are now certified. Then came licensure, and today having licensed social workers has become a requirement for every hospital.

That's what I hope will happen with community health workers. Social workers help people once they are in the hospital but the CHWs are the ones who make sure those people even make it to the hospital.

The next day, Karen introduced me to Maria, one of the community health workers who was completing her classes at Houston Community College for final certification. She was also a volunteer at

The Rose Galleria, our second location.

As a group, we made eleven visits to representatives' and senators' offices, mostly meeting with aides, walking the stairs from the fourth floor to the basement then to level two. We never stopped, except for a short break at lunch when no one was in their offices.

Our last appointment was with Lt. Governor Dewhurst. Six of us were scheduled for a photo op with him and we dutifully waited in the Senate Chamber. His aide kept apologizing, saying the Lt. Governor would be with us in five, then ten, then fifteen minutes. We waited. The official Capitol photographer was there, complete with his pink tie.

Finally, Lt. Gov. Dewhurst appeared. He is such a commanding figure, and with a height of six foot five, he towers over people. He greeted each person in our delegation, making note of where everyone was from, while the photographer, with the grace of much experience, gently moved us into place. We stood in front of the podium, the Lt. Gov. in the very middle, all of us framed by the Senate dais.

I continued to talk to him about our issues: CPRIT, BCCS, and patient navigators. It was obvious he was ready to excuse himself, when Maria stepped forward.

"I am a community health worker," she said, craning her neck to look up at him. "I was diagnosed with breast cancer in 2008. Even though I worked forty hours a week, I was not insured. I found help through The Rose. I would never have had treatment without The Rose. I know what it means to have a patient navigator help you through the process. My navigator was with me all the way, she was there to find my doctors, she made the appointments. I probably would have died without her."

She took a breath. "When I got well, I realized I had to do something to help other women, other women like me who didn't have insurance, find treatment. I quit my job of twelve years and went to Houston Community College for training."

To this day I don't know how she managed it, but in a split second a card appeared in her hand and she held it up at him. "This is my card. It shows I am a certified community health worker, and with it I can help women living anywhere in Texas get treatment."

His eyes remained on her as she finished her story; he looked down at his right arm and made a rubbing motion with his left hand. "That story gives me goose bumps. Tell me more about community health workers...patient navigators."

Maria glanced at me and I took it from there. I told him that every CHW had to obtain 160 classroom and clinical hours; that amount of training was not small and Texas was one of only three states to offer a formal certification for them.

He nodded. "What can we do, here in Austin, to help?" he asked.

"What we need is reimbursement," I said. "We need to implement CPT codes for reimbursement from insurance companies, Medicare, and Medicaid for CHW services. Without reimbursement they will never be used effectively." I added that Memorial Herman Health System had engaged patient navigators at their own expense in the emergency room and cardio units and saw a savings of nearly $2 million throughout the system.

I don't remember what else I said, I only remember him nodding.

Suddenly he raised both hands as if framing my body, and said, "In 32 seconds I have to be in a meeting with some people from the Senate Finance committee. It's an important group of people." Lord, I knew that. "Can you tell them, Senator Williams and Senator Hinojosa will be there and some others...can you tell them what you just told me in about eight sentences?"

"Absolutely!" I responded.

His hand clasped my arm and directed me to the conference room. Everything that happened next remains a blur. We entered the room and he apologized to the people sitting around the table for the delay. Ironically, I was speaking to the very senators I couldn't get an appointment with earlier that day. I launched into my spiel. I talked about community health workers, talked about the need to ensure that their services were reimbursed and their incredible importance to access to care. Too soon, my time was up.

An impeccably groomed woman gently ushered me out the door, and said, "You have no idea the good you just did for your cause." I thanked her and turned to my colleagues, their faces were expectant and all of them were smiling.

We managed to leave the Senate Chambers without embarrassing ourselves but we were on such a high that it would have been impossible not to notice this group of women, all wearing pink, were wildly ecstatic.

I hugged Maria, and exclaimed, "It was because of you!"

Karen was glowing, and affirmed, "That's right. They have to hear the story. Maria caught his attention with her story and Dorothy filled in the blanks. What a team."

By 3:30 in the afternoon, it was time to go home. I had agreed to drive four of the advocates back to Houston; it was a tight squeeze but we managed in my small SUV. Three women were crowded into the back seat, Maria next to one door, Robin in the middle, and the youngest in our group, Sylvia, nudged against the other door. Mary sat up front with me and, as women tend to do, we talked. The work in

Austin was behind us. Now we talked about our lives, our hopes, our worries.

We swapped stories about how we had met our husbands. I shared the abbreviated version of finding Patrick through the internet, about being fifty and how difficult the whole idea of dating was to me. I explained I had these rules concerning ever marrying again: The guy had to have a job; he couldn't live more than forty miles away; he couldn't come from a small town or only listen to Country Western music. I wouldn't date someone younger than me and he had to be "dynamite in bed." Everyone laughed.

I recounted how Patrick didn't fit all the criteria, being from Canada and loving Country Western and small towns. He did have a job, but darn it if he wasn't nine months younger than me! Another round of laughter filled the car.

Mary's voice was soft when she shared that it had been seven years since she had lost her love. "I might be ready to be with someone again, but since the mastectomy…" I knew the end of that sentence and had heard it so often over the years. Breast cancer may not change who we are on the inside but its impact on the body can be hell.

As we traveled those three hours together, we talked about the prejudice toward poverty and how it impacted women and their children the most. I told the story of my sister turning down a quarter an hour raise at a Dairy Queen because it would mean that her son, who had juvenile diabetes, would lose his Medicaid coverage, and she sure as heck could not afford his insulin. Everyone shared a similar story, citing some incident from their childhood or a time as an adult when they had seen that same prejudice or felt that distain.

We talked about the 51 community clinics that were about to close or reduce services, all because of the huge cuts in state funding for women's health. Shaking my head, I said, "And we all know that men are some of the primary users of those clinics. They go there for STD testing and treatment. How ironic."

Robin interjected, "Those same guys refuse to pay $6 for the treatment. I say to them, 'Come on, you can find six bucks. Don't go out there and infect your woman!'"

Something in her voice changed, it grew deeper, more serious. "Maybe what you're saying is right about poverty and prejudice, but I still remember the time when a Black person had to take the back door. I'm from Louisiana and it was bad growing up, still is in some places." She looked at the two women to each side of her, then said, "In fact, Ms. Dorothy, where I come from the only time you would ever see a white woman driving two Black women and two Hispanics around was if they worked for her."

It felt like someone had thrown a glass of water in my face.

"Really?" I responded, my tone incredulous. That thought would never have occurred to me.

"Yes, really! I'm only 57, and yet those things happened in my lifetime, I can remember those times."

Mary nodded and so did Maria. My mind raced, tossing around the implications that statement held.

Here we were, five women coming back from a day of advocacy, all of us speaking up for a change in laws, a day when we were more separated by who was a survivor and who was not than by the color of our skin.

Everyone was quiet for a long time. Finally, I said, "I think the real reason I am so adamant about the importance of CHWs is because it is a way for women to get a really good job. I'm talking about regular women, women who didn't have a chance to go to college, women who are street savvy and smart, especially women who speak different languages. It's a way to actually have a career. CHW training gives them a chance." Everyone agreed.

We arrived in Houston, tired but still talking. I dropped each one off near their cars. We all hugged and said goodbye. Maria was the last one.

She said, "Thank you, Dorothy. I loved your stories; it was so good to meet you. Thank you for bringing us back."

I said, "No problem." Then I asked, "Maria, I've been meaning to ask you. Who was your navigator?" I couldn't remember who was on the team in 2008. "You said she was so good to you. Was it Monica?"

"She was good to me, helped me so much." She stressed the words good and help.

"But it wasn't Monica?" I asked again.

"No," she shook her head, and said softly, "It was Lynn."

I felt that familiar rock of sadness lodged behind my heart crumble a bit, and in a clear voice I said, "Lynn was a very good patient navigator."

She nodded, "Yes, she was." Her gaze was direct, her meaning clear. She turned and walked to her car. A few months later, we would hire Maria. She'd be part of the navigation team that moves hundreds of women into treatment each year.

I left the parking lot thinking about the five women, each heading off in opposite directions, going to their own homes. All of us were different, but for those hours we spent together and the stories we shared, we were all the same.

Chapter 29
Vicky's Story

Throughout the history of The Rose, many stories have made me cry, but none quite like Vicky's. I first met Vicky in 2002 at the Federation of Houston Professional Women's annual event. Vicky was busy coordinating some part of the Federation's Women of Excellence award event that honored forty women from different organizations. I was one of the recipients.

Two years later, in 2004, I ran into Vicky again. I should have sensed the signs of trouble. When I saw her, she offhandedly said she needed to come to The Rose for a mammogram. I told her to call the office and that we could probably work her in soon. A couple of months passed and we met again at another fundraising event.

I don't remember much about the event. I only remember Vicky sitting at the reception table, greeting everyone as they entered and chatting away—her smile ever present. When she saw me, her face clouded and almost immediately after saying hi, she said she needed to call for a mammogram appointment. Something cold moved through my veins. I paused and really looked at her. She was staring down at the RSVP list, pen in hand, absorbed by the list. She was a small woman and her tiny frame was gobbled up by the big chair.

"Vicky?" I asked, "Is there something going on?" It wasn't exactly the most diplomatic question, considering the crowd streaming by.

But she met my eyes and said, "Yes." After a pause, she added, "It has been a couple of months."

"And you didn't call us?" I asked, wanting to scream.

"I was waiting until I had the money," she explained, her voice dropping. "Since Jay was laid off, we haven't had insurance."

I was confused. I couldn't understand why she hadn't called us. Almost simultaneously, my mind was calculating how soon we could get her in. I dug my cell phone out of my purse and started to call the office. She reached out and her fingers closed over my phone to stop me. "I promise I'll call." Her smile had returned, "Honest, just let me finish this luncheon."

"Are you absolutely sure? I'll check when I get back to the office. I know we can get you in soon."

Within a week, Vicky came for her appointment, but she refused to accept financial assistance, insisting on paying for her diagnostic mammogram and ultrasound work-up. By the time we got her to biopsy, it was obvious that she would need to go through one of our programs.

Vicky's cancer wasn't small and its location wasn't good. It was an aggressive tumor that would need equally aggressive treatment. After it was all said and done, she qualified for the state program. She had been eligible for it all along, right from the very beginning. She began her treatment and had surgery, but with every step forward there was a step back. She had simply waited too long. At the height of her treatment, her husband Jay was diagnosed with cancer as well. Months later, he lost his battle.

That's when we learned that Vicky would be on chemotherapy for the rest of her life. Through it all she never lost her smile, her zest for life, her kindness or her willingness to be a support for anyone else diagnosed with cancer. She was always the first woman we called to talk to a newly diagnosed woman, the first to volunteer for any event, and the first to share her story—including her delay.

Even though Vicky knew about The Rose, she had been reluctant to use the sponsorship program because, she said, "I didn't want to take the spot of someone else who might need the help more." She was like so many others, a woman not used to asking for charity, proud, accustomed to paying her own way. Realizing why Vicky had put off making an appointment weighed heavily on my heart.

Eight years later, in 2012, Vicky and I met at a local tea room to talk. The air conditioning was barely working, struggling to combat Houston's July heat and humidity. In spite of all I knew about Vicky the patient, I didn't really know much about Vicky the person. I wanted to know her better, before it was too late.

Her dark indigo eyes stared into me and her face seemed as fragile as a piece of ancient pottery. Her pale skin made the reddish rim of her naked eyelids stand out and the ridge meant for eyebrows was stark in its bareness.

"How many treatments? How many years has it been now?" I asked

"Let's see..." she said, holding up her left hand and counting on tiny, childlike fingers, "Taxol, Taxotere, Adriamycin, Cytoxin, Zolada, Tykerb, Exempra, Herceptin... there's one other." She paused and smiled at me, "My hair actually starting growing back when I was on Taxol. I was diagnosed in 2004 and on chemotherapy for a year. Then, nearly three years later, it came back and had metastasized in my bones. I've been on some kind of 'cocktail' ever since."

Those cocktails, a combination of chemotherapy drugs usually administered intravenously over several hours, meant a chance, maybe her only chance, at life.

For some women, breast cancer means a six to eight month bout with chemotherapy, radiation, or both, and usually some kind of surgery. Yet after a time, which assuredly feels like forever, they are pronounced cancer free. They go on with their lives, dreading the annual examination, but with each passing year, survival becomes more and more of a reality.

Other women lose the battle way too soon after diagnosis because the cancer is late stage or super aggressive and has already started its raging destruction through the body, encompassing too many vital organs before the chemotherapy even has a chance.

For some, the cancer seemingly responds to treatment, appears gone and then without any warning comes back with a vengeance.

Vicky's cancer fell somewhere between all those scenarios. At the time she was diagnosed, she was the sole support of her family, taking on every possible client to keep her accounting business going and to keep the wolf away from the door. Vicky didn't make enough to pay the exorbitant costs of Cobra insurance after her husband was laid off and she could not afford private insurance. She didn't think they were poor enough to qualify for public health; not that she would have known how that system worked anyway.

"I knew something was wrong," she said, her voice almost childlike. "I could feel the lump in my breast but it would get bigger and then smaller, so I convinced myself it was just the stress. I knew cancer didn't come and go. I had plenty to be stressed about. I was in a job I didn't like, working full time and then going home at night and spending hours doing bookkeeping for my clients. I was building my business, one small account at a time. My work was all we had. I didn't have time to worry about anything else."

"After a while, though, the area didn't go down, it grew. Then I noticed the orange peel on my skin. I knew it was cancer." Her blue eyes were searching, staring out over the space beyond our table. For a moment she was somewhere else, the essence of her being had disappeared to some distant place, locked in another time.

Eventually, she turned her head toward me and looked me directly in the eyes. "Breast cancer has been like an adventure for me." Her words caught me off-guard. She pushed at the brim of her baseball cap, moving it up and a little off her forehead as tiny beads of sweat glistened on her skin.

"An adventure?" I asked, "I've heard some women call it a gift or journey, but for you it's been an adventure? "

"In college," she said, "I wanted to be a nurse and had started clinical training. So when I got sick, I was intrigued learning the different ways each chemical or combination of chemicals interacted with the body, the side effects they could cause and how they worked. I knew going into my treatments pretty much what to expect," she said, with a matter of fact shrug of her shoulders.

"That knowing was important to me. I had to get a handle on the things I could control and learn how to let go of the things I could not control. I have had a lot of chemotherapy just to stay alive. At least until the cancer gets smart again and stops responding to whatever regimen I'm on. Then we find another cocktail and start over."

I marveled at her matter of fact attitude. I knew that even when she wasn't battling the effects of chemotherapy, she was fighting an infection or having another 'spot' appear that needed more tests and weeks of waiting for results. One of the infections had settled in her jawbone, and required her taking antibiotics every four hours, every day for six weeks.

She could live without ever having hair again, or eyebrows, or eyelashes, but I wondered how she managed the day in and day out of simply getting through the basics, always being at the door of exhaustion, knowing the cancer would never be cured. No matter what, cancer is cancer, better treatments don't necessarily equate to a better journey.

"After eight years, what is my purpose now?" Her eyes seemed even wider, set deeper as she looked up at me from under the cap's brim. "To still be alive when so many others have died makes me wonder." Her voice was soft.

"But Vicky, think of all the people who have turned to you and asked you to talk with their friend or family member. Isn't that a part of your purpose?" I argued.

She shrugged. Her lower lip trembled ever so slightly. I cringed at the feebleness of my words.

I asked, "What is it you find yourself sharing with perfect strangers anyway?"

"It depends on where they are in their diagnosis or treatment," she said, a look of concentration on her face. "Most people just need someone to listen to them. I tell them that this is their journey, not mine, not their spouses, and not their best friend's. I try to help them know how to educate themselves, know what to ask the doctor, and beyond that to feel like they have some control."

"Control?" I asked. She was using that word again. I knew that of all the losses of the cancer journey, being stripped of control tops the list. I ticked the items off in my mind: the loss of a breast; the loss of hair; loss of privacy as yet another doctor or tech inspects her body; plus the financial losses and for many even losing the ability to make a living. The most tragic seemed to be losing the support of a spouse or suddenly realizing friends don't come around anymore. Of course, the ultimate loss, the one no one ever wants to discuss, is losing one's life. To me, the onlooker, a lay person, a non-survivor, there just wasn't much left within a patient's control.

"Control!" Vicky replied firmly, her soothing voice supported by her measured and methodical cadence. "I admit that it has been a hard one for me, but my friend Pat really put me straight on it. She said, 'Look, Vicky, there are things you can't control. You won't be able to control the appointments or the number of hours it takes for chemotherapy, you can't control how good you'll feel those days after infusions, but you can control the amount of work you do that week. You can't control when your hair will fall out, so decide when. Set a date and have it shaved off. You can make sure you are around positive people and folks who support you. You can control what you eat.'" Vicky laughed, "Anytime I found myself getting off on the wrong track Pat would haul me back to the right one."

"Having good friends is important," I smiled, "especially…"

"…those that allow you to have a 24 hour pity party," she interrupted, nodding her head. "For 24 hours, I'm allowed to feel sorry for myself—to have a pity party. I encourage the people I talk to to do the same. There's something good about knowing you can wallow in it for at least 24 hours, complain, cry, rage against the unfairness of it all, feel as low as you want to." She grinned, "I usually don't need the whole 24 hours anymore. But if I do, I take it. Then I can move on."

Too soon our visit was over and it was time for me to leave. We hugged. I was startled to find that her body was just skin and bones, one of my arms could wrap around her entire frame. Her hands in mine were almost weightless. When I glanced back to wave goodbye I saw that she had sat back down at the table; her shoulders were not so square, her cap was pushed back on her forehead. She stared into the cup sitting before her.

I quickly turned my face away. Once again, I cried.

I guess you really don't know someone until you hear her friends describe her, especially if that talk happens around her death bed. When Vicky became gravely ill, three of her best women friends took turns being with her. Through the last months of her life, those three spent chunks of time with her.

It was a Friday morning when Vicky couldn't stand up. Carolyn was with her. The call to Dr. Haq ended with one instruction: Take her to the hospital.

Vicky had made everyone promise that they would let her die at home, in her own bed, with her cats. Carolyn said, "If we go to the hospital…"

Vicky finished the sentence, "…I probably won't ever come home again."

So they declined making that last trip to the hospital. Dr. Haq came to the apartment around noon and ordered hospice at home. The nurse arrived, morphine in hand, and the watch began.

On her last weekend there was a revolving door of friends coming in and out, telling stories, sharing memories, signing the Vicky book, sharing a last wish or thought, singing to her. Vicky was still alert and awake. But early Monday morning there was a shift; soon she was drifting in and out of a comatose state, sometimes responding to questions, sometimes not.

At noon that day, Myrleen sent me an email: "Vicky is unresponsive. My heart is breaking."

The journey down south on I-45 was a long thirty minutes and I prayed I wasn't too late. Seeing her tiny shriveled body on the bed didn't alarm me, I had visited with her the weekend before when she was in the hospital. But without her snug fitting cap, the scraps of fuzz on her scalp stood out, defiant reminders of hair long gone. Her face was drawn, the skin stretched over bones that stood out too sharply.

Her eyes were closed and the tiny oxygen hoses that looped around each ear and came together to meet at her nose emphasized the hollow space at her temples. That space seemed to deepen the longer I looked at her. I searched for any sign of recognition from her when I spoke. There was none.

I sat alone with her for a long time, holding her hand under the covers. In spite of the drone of the huge television that perched on the chest of drawers at the end of her bed, the long silences between her breaths dominated the room. I pulled the blanket up over her shoulders, hiding her jutting collarbones covered only by the slimmest trace of skin.

I soon became lost in memories of all the times Vicky had volunteered for The Rose. I remembered a pre-cancer Vicky, smiling, tossing balls during a Rose fundraiser. Then I saw a post-cancer Vicky, wearing her wig, speaking to a crowd, sharing her story.

Other scenes floated through my mind. One by one, the memories continued: her playing the ukulele at the Shrimp Boil; Vicky in remission and on a cruise ship showing us how to dance down and dirty to the twist; a very bald Vicky wearing her pink Santa hat and ever-present smile at her surprise fifty-fifth birthday party in December. She was so achingly thin; the mask of death had already crept onto her face.

Vicky said The Rose gave her eight more years; time she was convinced she never would have had if she had gone through the public health system. She said with a prognosis of advanced cancer, she would have been dead in ten months.

Not our program, but her incredible will to live, I thought.

Noises were coming from the living room and I heard people walking toward the bedroom. As they gathered around Vicky's bed, their talk became light and happy, recounting their lunch experience to her, telling her of the God awful long wait, the mediocre food. But Vicky never stirred. Her breath had dropped to two respirations a minute. They drew closer to her, one sat beside her, another at the end of the bed, each reached out to touch some part of her body, stroking her leg or patting her arm or gently rubbing her forehead.

One woman said softly, "You remember that Vicky said she wanted this done by Monday night." Heads nodded. The clock on the wall marked the time: 5:33 p.m.

After we moved to the living room, her friends shared one last story about Vicky.

"Vicky went into hospice on Friday, and all through Saturday she was alert and able to talk with us. But by Sunday it was obvious she was deteriorating, it was harder to rouse her and she was sleeping more. Her priest was out of town and would not be able to visit until late Monday. We were worried that she wouldn't make it until Monday, so we found another priest to come and perform last rites.

"As we all gathered around her bed and the priest was about to start, Vicky held up her hand, motioning the folks at the end of the bed standing in front of the television set to move to one side. She said clearly, 'Could we wait a minute? The NASCAR race is about to start and I really want to see Danica Patrick, the first female racer to ever make the cut, take off!'"

Only Vicky would have stopped her own last rites for one final moment of absorbing life.

Two days later, Vicky went to heaven.

Life at The Rose continues. Volunteers organize fundraisers, willingly giving their time and talents. More grants are researched, case statements written, proposals submitted. Letters to donors mailed, phone calls made.

We'll ask, beg, rebound from rejections, and celebrate successes.

We'll do whatever it takes to bring in even one more dollar. Because we are certain there will be so many other women, just like Vicky, we have yet to serve.

Chapter 30
Camera Shy

"The film crew will be at The Rose by 6:15 a.m.; first they will film the doctor, then do facility shots at 7; you'll be on live at 8 a.m. Be there by 7:30." Karen's email was to the point: who, what, where, when—her instructions concise, clear, and most of all, not to be ignored.

As soon as I walked through the automatic sliding glass doors of the building, the familiar sight of the over-bright lights flooded the lobby. Immediately to my right, Andrea Watkins, news reporter for a local television station, was interviewing our physician. To my left, Karen waited.

Andrea had just completed her own year-long bout with breast cancer and its treatment. During this telecast she was showing off her hair, short blond waves surrounded her face. It was her own hair, and she and the anchor at the station bantered about it during the live telecast. Andrea had been very public about her diagnosis, allowing television cameras to follow her through the treatment and procedures. After months of wearing wigs on air, it probably wouldn't have mattered how short or how unruly her locks were; they were her own.

Soon it was time for my live interview. As the cameraman repositioned the camera, Andrea turned to me. "This is what I want to go over with you," she said, scanning the tablet in her hand, clicking off the subjects. "But I really want you to talk about your part in starting The Rose." Andrea looked at me pointedly.

I glanced over at Karen. She cocked her head and stared at me, eyes unblinking, feigned innocence covered her face as she silently asked, *Isn't it time to tell your story?* Even working only part time with us, Karen knew more about me than any other staff member.

Karen had an appealing and genuine manner, her short red hair with sometime highlights of brown or blond emphasized the smattering of freckles that covered her face, giving her a forever youthful appearance. She seemed totally approachable, had a natural gift of gab and was sharp as a tack. She had an uncanny knack of generating provocative conversations between people and organizations.

She knew her stuff and never missed an opportunity to promote The Rose in whatever way possible and using whatever vehicle available. She was a whiz at social media, made our Facebook page sing, and she could whip out a news release faster than the sharp shooters of the Old West could brandish their side arms. Today's filming was the result of one of her media efforts.

Andrea didn't miss the exchange between Karen and me.

Karen responded in her most professional sounding voice. "Dorothy doesn't usually tell her story, but actually she has a very personal reason of her own for being so determined to help women."

I tossed her a you-better-stop-before-I-kill-you look, smiling sweetly before turning back to talk with Andrea. She raised her left hand, motioning me to stop as her right hand moved to the earpiece; she was occupied listening to instructions from the mother station.

I stood up and walked over to Karen. "I don't see any point..." I whispered.

"It's up to you," Karen interrupted. She studied a fingernail before looking up at me and pointing that same finger at me. "But I'm here to tell you that your story is powerful. Remember the other day at the Women's Health Initiative meeting? All those women were ready to discount you and what you said because <u>they</u> figured you were just another out of touch wealthy woman, someone who always had money and power and influence. When <u>they</u> heard your story, <u>they</u> were the ones who said, 'She knows what we're fighting; she's the face of the women we are working for!'" Her finger punched the air each time she said the word 'they.' "But like I said, it's totally up to you." She returned to studying her hand.

Right, I thought. Karen had been pushing me to share my story for a long time. My stomach was doing flip flops. *Tell my story? Why? What good would it do?*

Andrea's voice broke into my internal debate. "So, what is your story?"

I slowly moved to camera position, my thoughts racing, wondering how to frame my response. Andrea waited, her gaze was direct.

"My mother died when I was young, she was uninsured. She was a single mother, worked hard, but there weren't any services for her. Every time I see that frightened look in the eyes of one of our uninsured women, I see my mother."

I'll never forget that look—it was the same look I have seen in a wounded animal, the creature that is too hurt to know where to turn and too scared to trust anyone.

The irony of my mother's story was she worked as a housekeeper in a large hospital. Every day as she was mopping floors, around her walked the very people—the doctors, nurses, medical folks—who could have diagnosed her. But of course, she wouldn't have bothered them, not in her position.

Without insurance, she waited, way too long. I was there when the surgeon explained, "We opened her up. The cancer was everywhere so we closed her up. She doesn't have long to live."

Back then, no one mentioned the word cancer. People actually thought it was contagious. My aunt was furious with me for telling my mother what the doctors found. I didn't care. My mother deserved to know the truth. She deserved so much more from life. Almost six months later, I held her hand when cancer stole her final breath.

The cameraman called out, lights were in position. Andrea nodded and the interview began. She spelled my name, paused, nodded her head, then added CEO and co-founder.

No fig leaf shots, I reminded myself silently, unclasping my hands in front of me. *Stand up tall. Stop making those fists,* I ordered my errant hands. *Breathe, smile, remember this is live, no retakes.* I ticked each instruction off in my brain. I waited through that incredibly familiar and long period of time until, finally, the reporter cued that the camera was rolling.

"I'm here today with Dorothy Gibbons, co-founder of The Rose." Andrea moved through the interview with the ease of a seasoned reporter and led me through explaining the range of services and the impact of insured women coming to us. I ticked off the answers, hoping I hadn't forgotten something important.

"Why did you start The Rose? What has it been now, 26 years ago?"

"Yes. In the mid-'80s, women didn't know about mammography, and the times were a lot like today, too many people without insurance." I launched into my standard, albeit shortest version of our beginnings.

"But for you it was personal," Andrea said, the invitation was clear.

I stared back at her, nodding in agreement, trusting that my smile concealed the horror I felt. My throat tightened.

"Very personal?" she continued, waiting for my reply. I knew I had to respond, unfilled seconds on live camera were like hours to the viewer, and it was obvious she wasn't going to let me skip this question.

Maybe, just maybe, I don't want to...skirt it, avoid it...any longer. The thought pushed through the mounting waves of anxiety flooding my body. My words, hesitant at first, draped with a huskiness that alarmed me, seemed to be coming from some distant place inside me that had been held in check too long. "Yes, it was. Very personal." Suddenly I was 22 years old again, standing beside the hospital bed, watching the wasted body of my mother, hearing her ragged breath, seeing that look in her eyes and feeling very helpless. Tears sprang to my eyes.

"My mother died when I was in my early twenties, she was in a charity hospital." The words climbed out, some seized by the choking in my throat, but thank goodness they were audible. "She was a single mother of four children, she worked hard. Even then I wondered what would have been different in her life if she'd had insurance."

I paused for the briefest space in time. "I've seen what happens to a family when their Mama isn't around to keep things together." The waves inside me slowly subsided, the images from over forty years ago faded.

My voice grew stronger. "For her type of cancer there wasn't a place that could help her. But today The Rose exists and there is no reason, absolutely no reason, any woman should die of breast cancer because she can't afford a mammogram."

"Thank you." Andrea reached over to me, "I know that wasn't easy to share." She hugged me with one arm, pulling my rigid body toward her.

It was the first time I had told my story on camera, and it would be one of the few times I ever did share it publicly. In my mind, there would always be too many other stories about the women of The Rose that needed telling.

Later I returned to the office to check emails. Karen heard my gasp. I turned the monitor toward her so she could read the email I had just received from Yvette, our phone attendant.

It said that while I was on TV a lady had called in and was in tears. She said that I was telling the story about my mother with cancer and her being a single mother. She said it touched her heart because she herself was a single mother and had a daughter and son, and she didn't want to put her kids through that same struggle. She was already 48 and had never had a mammogram because she never made time for it and mainly she was scared to get one. But she called to make an appointment, saying she was "doing it for her kids."

A smile danced around Karen's mouth as she looked at me and said a single word, "See?"

Chapter 31
A Color or a Cause

Over the years the color pink and the pink ribbon have become synonymous with breast cancer. For some the ribbon is a symbol of camaraderie, for others who are battling the disease that same symbol is despised and avoided at all costs. For some women that magical five-year survival mark is the time to pack away the pink, hoping that they never have reason to wear one of those ribbons again. For others the pink paraphernalia is resurrected once a year to be worn proudly during a walk or run fundraiser. That's enough, no analysis needed, just wear it once a year.

I wonder if Estée Lauder ever imagined the worldwide impact of her gift of the pink ribbon. Legend has it that she was the first to use the pink ribbon in a marketing campaign that connected it to breast cancer and then literally gave the idea away. A different version of the ribbon's creation attributes it to another woman who asked that it not be used for sales.

Who could have predicted in the 1980s that breast cancer would reach an epidemic level? Who knew that the day would come when breast cancer would need its own banner; something to unify the growing masses of diagnosed women, reluctant recruits to a group that no one would voluntarily join?

Someone once told me the symbol drove her crazy. "That ribbon is an incomplete infinity sign," she argued, "it is waiting for someone or something to close the loop and stop the madness of this disease." To her, leaving the ribbon open meant, at least metaphorically, inviting in an endless loss of life and an endless time of searching for a cure.

The coupling of the color pink with breast cancer does seem to make strange bed partners. Pink, the color of sweetness and little girls, is supposed to have a soothing effect, yet the women I know who wear the ribbon are anything but calm.

In the end, the meaning of the pink ribbons can only be defined by the woman or man going through the disease. I asked a handful of women, from different walks of life, at different stages in recovery, "What does the pink ribbon mean to you? Is it something you wear? Something you like to receive as a gift, something you like to see?"

Sandra, who was over five years out, said, "Pink ribbon gifts are good in moderation. I went through many different moods during the first few years after diagnosis. I remember, at times, thinking if I saw one more pink ribbon I would scream, but I am over that now."

Cecilia, a colleague who also worked in non-profits, was pretty adamant. "I've gotten pink ribbons and/or pink beribboned objects from folks who want to celebrate my heroism/survival. That's very sweet and I appreciate the thought, but for some reason, it pisses me off at times. It seemed like I was suffocated in pink ribbons and by the word "survivor"...pink pink pink or survivor survivor survivor...It seemed that my whole identity had become consumed by breast cancer, and that's the exact opposite of what I wanted. Yes, my life had been dramatically affected, but I wanted to take the lessons I learned from my two experiences and LIVE...FULLY. And MOVE ON. It seemed that suddenly I had pink ribbons wrapped around my ankles like Marley's ghost from *A Christmas Carol*."

She took a breath before adding, "I'd rather the pink ribbon became something more aggressive. I don't want to be associated with a soft, frilly, feminine pink ribbon that says "Yay, I survived and can go on and be a sweet woman the world can embrace." If I wear a pink ribbon, I want it to have jagged edges, blood on the cuts and scars representing the ripped families, the lost mothers, the lost libido, the stripped femininity, the evisceration that so many of us go through with this experience. If you want to show heroism, then it's not going to be a nursery pink!"

Marian had a different take on the ribbon, and told me, "The pink ribbon gives me hope and assurance that there are people out there willing to work for a cure for breast cancer. It gives me comfort. I love to receive gifts with the pink ribbon on them. I like it when people ask me about my breast cancer because I know that this is something that I will fight every day for the rest of my life. I want to help other women fight too. I plan to live every day to the fullest and get every delicious drop out of life, and the pink ribbon is on the front of my shield!"

And so the jury remains out, at least for me. Gift it or not, disliked or not, it still represents a disease no one would volunteer to endure. My unscientific research provided nothing definite. The debate about wearing, giving, displaying the pink ribbon is fraught with emotion. But I wonder, is pink just a color, or is it truly a cause? Probably a bit of both.

When I see a woman or man wearing one, I know somewhere there is a connection to the many hundreds of women I've known. I have to wonder if their connection involves a woman rejoicing in recovery or—like the ones I've cried with—those who did not.

To me it means what it was meant to—awareness. It means we can talk about a subject that no one wanted to touch in the '80s and one that is still taboo in parts of the world.

It means a high school senior inspiring her classmates to buy 500 pink tee-shirts, which raised $10,000 in honor of her mother who was battling breast cancer. It means seeing firefighters wearing pink helmets, walking up and down the street to raise money for mammograms. It means selling pink cupcakes or handmade bracelets made from pink cords or quilts covered in pink squares of fabric—all because someone took the time to honor or remember a loved one.

And, more than once, seeing the pink ribbon has meant a woman admitting that she needs a mammogram but she doesn't have a lot of money to pay for it or insurance to cover it.

That's when the color pink makes the difference. That's when she finds The Rose.

Chapter 32
Too Young for a Mammogram

The two gentlemen sitting across the conference room table from me were well dressed and had a certain air of graciousness about them. From the opening pleasantries I knew they were both retired, yet very active in hobbies and their church. They were visiting The Rose, doing an on-site visit and gathering information to take back to the larger grants review committee.

"My wife used to come to The Rose. She had a scare and is now at MD Anderson. When I told her where I was going today, she had nothing but praise for your organization. She said you had the best equipment." John had performed a lot of site visits to non-profit organizations; he had visited us once before, many years ago.

"That's because of the generosity of groups like yours, who make sure our equipment is always state of the art." I smiled, thankful the meeting was starting off on such a good note.

He looked at his colleague. "Yes, I am familiar with The Rose. Our church has funded their programs for years. They do wonderful work." Then he addressed me. "But with your budget, I don't see how our grant of $10,000 will have much impact."

Trina assured me later that neither men saw my visceral reaction, "It was barely noticeable, Dorothy. But for a moment I was afraid you were going to reach over the table and shake him!" she laughed.

Ironically, my one concern for this visit was about the small number of women that $10,000 would help. I feared they would think that 25 women weren't enough, but then we're talking about covering the costs of providing pretty sophisticated medical services, not bags of groceries. I was totally prepared to explain the complexities of the procedures involved for each of those women, diagnostic mammogram, followed by an ultrasound, both with a physical examination and the physician present to determine next steps.

After what seemed a short eternity, I found my voice and

recovered. "John, our request is for services for young women, for women who are under forty years old. Believe me, there isn't any area where your gift could make a bigger impact."

He frowned. "I don't understand."

"There is absolutely no funding available for women under forty. There was a time when we could apply some of the state funds to that age group, but the criteria changed in January. For the past three months we have had sixty to seventy young women who need services on a waiting list. We really count on grants from independent organizations such as your church for those women," I responded, but I could tell I wasn't making the most compelling case.

"Let me tell you about Sasha, who was only 31 years old when diagnosed. In fact, I'll show you a short video and let her share her own story." It only took a few seconds to turn on the overhead projector, and soon, Sasha's face was filling up the screen.

"When I found my lump, it was late one evening. I had just put my two kids to bed. I was exhausted and turned on the TV. For some reason I put my hand on my chest, and call it God or Angels or whatever, my hand went right to the lump. I knew it wasn't good. I had watched my mother go through breast cancer. All I could think about were my little ones, my baby was only a year old, and who would take care of them. I didn't think the night would ever end. I couldn't wait to get it checked."

Sasha was stunningly beautiful and genuine. Even over a video, her big brown eyes conveyed the depth of her fear. Tears spilled over, and she said, "But no one would see me. We were facing some rough times, and I let my insurance drop. I kept it for the kids of course, but thought I could get by for a few months. Besides being uninsured, I kept being told I was too young for a mammogram. I couldn't get anyone to pay attention, let alone take me seriously.

"That's when I remembered that my mother had gone to The Rose five years earlier when she didn't have insurance and needed services. I found my lump on a Tuesday, it was on a Wednesday when I called, they saw me on a Friday and had me back in for a biopsy by Tuesday of the next week. I knew it was cancer. I told my mother, 'When that pathology comes back we're going shopping.' I was determined not to let it beat me!"

"But that's not Sasha's entire story," I said, turning to the two men. "The Rose navigated her into treatment and she has done well. It would be enough knowing that she's going to be alive to raise her boys. But she went further. After her chemotherapy started and her hair fell out, she tried to find a place that sold wigs that were cute and comfortable and offered underwear that was attractive. She wanted to look like and feel like the young woman she was. She went to a few shops but everything was for older women. She said, 'The bras were awful, the wigs were short, every time I went into one of those stores I came out feeling even more depressed.'

"So she promised herself that when she finished treatment, she was going to do something for young women. She borrowed money, found the perfect location, filled it with beautiful underclothes and wigs. Tomorrow they celebrate the first year anniversary of Cure and Company. It has become the 'go to' place for young women with breast cancer. Sasha is an esthetician and she knows how to take care of skin. She carries special lotions for skin that has been damaged due to radiation; she does facials and fixes eyebrows. Most of all, she understands and is able to show women who are in treatment how to look good. She's making a difference in the lives of so many young women.

"We were able to serve Sasha because of grants like this one. She didn't have the money for a diagnostic work-up. Four hundred dollars—that's all that was standing between her and a diagnosis. Every year, 3,000 young women turn to us for help. A delay in service for any one of them could have disastrous results. Believe me, this $10,000 will have a huge impact, it could mean a young woman's life!"

I could have told him hundreds of stories. Not all of them had happy endings. Breast cancer can be so aggressive in young women.

John assured me that he would recommend our proposal be funded, and added, "But the decision won't be made until November and it is June." He grimaced and kind of shrugged his shoulders.

"I understand. There will be just as much need then." I smiled, inviting them to take a tour with me. They would see young women in our reception area; they would hear other stories from our patient navigators.

We wouldn't share the case we had had that week, it was too sad. A woman, mother of twins, had to make the hard decision about the unborn babies, another set of twins, she carried. At only 28, her chemotherapy would need to be as aggressive as her cancer. Not a good scenario.

We did share the story of another uninsured young woman who was diagnosed and navigated the previous year. She had gone through her pregnancy while having surgery and a full range of chemotherapy. Only two weeks ago, we'd seen Kay and her eight-month-old, incredibly healthy baby boy. She was one of six Women of The Rose that we featured for the Bikers Against Breast Cancer event. There was something so poignant about seeing her holding her baby against her chest, his precious little body filling up the space where her left breast had been.

Someday I hope we will be able to screen any woman, regardless of her age. We MUST do away with the illusionary standard that screening is not valuable for young women, especially those who are under forty years old! Nothing magically happens to a woman's body at forty or fifty or any age that makes it ready for screening.

In February, 2013, the headline screamed, "Study Sees More Breast Cancer at Young Age." The accompanying story explained that statistics showed that the number of women aged 25 to 39 with advanced breast cancer had increased over the last thirty years. I will never understand why there has to be a study to prove something we've known for years.

Young women continue to be the most medically underserved population we see at The Rose. It doesn't matter if she is Black, white, Hispanic, or Asian. It makes no difference if she is insured or uninsured. If a woman is under forty years old, she will face tremendous barriers in finding breast care. And if she can't find care, the cancer will grow, and at a far more rapid rate than in older women, and the race against time will be lost.

But I know that changing the screening age, at least in my lifetime, would take a true miracle. First it would require that the medical community find a way to screen young women that is 'cost effective.' (Forget the cost of treatment for late stage cancer or the price paid when another young woman dies before her kids get to middle school.)

And those procedures would need to be considered screening and fall under preventative healthcare with 100% coverage. No longer would a young woman be penalized by calling it a diagnostic procedure, which would require her to pay against deductibles or copays (if she's lucky enough to be insured).

Once the official recommendations include younger women, a process that will require years, then attending physicians, who have much too much to remember already, will have to adopt them. The change will need help from all major media outlets to generate positive awareness that will empower women to be proactive about their bodies.

Providing mammography screening regardless of age? It's an idea almost as crazy as providing screening regardless of the ability to pay.

Chapter 33
Pink October

The rain pelted down as I walked out of the house at 4:15 a.m. It was dark and the wind whipped around me, threatening to sweep away the bags in my hands and making havoc of my carefully arranged hair. I was headed to Sugarland for the first 5:15 a.m. live television spot that would kick off the month of October and highlight the Susan G. Komen Houston Race for the Cure. The TV producer wanted folks from The Rose to add to the crowd, and Karen had convinced her that our new mobile mammography unit would be a perfect backdrop! As it turned out, it sure was.

The first thing I saw as I pulled up was the Channel 2 mobile van, with its fifteen foot tall satellite extension reaching into the sky. Huge canisters of lights brightened the walkway and fat lengths of black wire snaked along the ground and sidewalk. Yep, the media was ready.

The second thing I saw was a sea of pink. At least fifty people were moving in and out of the fitness studio, all dressed in pink. The costumes were outrageous. One woman announced she bought her sequined pink high-heeled boots for her sixtieth birthday and her sixteenth year as a survivor. Others had on pink shirts and shorts, but Diane stole the show in her pink organza tutu and cut-off survivor-pink tee-shirt. Even the men were decked out in pink cowboy hats, pink vests, and oversized pink sunglasses.

The crowd was jazzed. Ruben, the early morning on-the-road, mostly crazy and fun TV reporter kept the energy high. He teased the women about their pink hair until some turned even pinker from blushing. Then he'd turn to a survivor, and in the most caring way, he'd ask what the Race meant to her. He lingered with Marisol, a young woman who was diagnosed by The Rose and had been selected as one of the 2014 Faces of Komen.

The camera rolled on, filming some segments inside the fitness studio and of the crowd standing in front of our shiny new mobile unit. No one there knew it, but the fact that The Rose now had a fourth mobile unit was nothing short of a miracle in itself.

Only five weeks before, Kim Marling, executive director of the Woodforest Charitable Foundation, had called me. She and husband Robert, owners of the Woodforest National Banks, had created the foundation and their charity work extended throughout several states. Last year, their support of our golf tournament was significant and had been part of the $95,000 we had raised toward the fourth mobile van.

When she called around 8 a.m., her questions caught me off-guard. "Dorothy, how much is left to be raised for the new mobile unit?" She paused, "What would it take to be able to order it and get it on the road?"

Thinking that she was soliciting new supporters for this year's golf tournament, I told her we had raised about a third of it and there was a sizable chunk remaining.

"Exactly how much do you need?" It was obvious Kim was on her mobile phone, but what I didn't know until well into the conversation was that she was actually headed to her own annual mammography appointment. Ask any survivor about the anxiety they feel when going for their annual examination, yet I never would have guessed what was going on in Kim's mind.

I said I could get that exact figure and be back with her ASAP.

"Dorothy, we really do need a unit for the women here in Montgomery County. If you had a fourth unit, could it primarily serve this area?"

I said yes. There was no dearth of uninsured in Montgomery County.

Her next statement left me speechless. "Then go ahead and order it. The foundation will make up the difference. Just let me know how much you need to pay off—exactly how much."

Five weeks later, there I was, standing in front of the unit proudly bearing Woodforest Charitable Foundation's logo, with my mobile staff, Ashlyn and Lilia, who beamed as I talked into the camera.

Once the filming was done, I raced home to fix my rain-beaten hair and change from my Rose tee-shirt into my business best. I headed to the office. It was 8:30 a.m. On my way I dropped off my two pink jackets at the cleaners, kicking myself that I hadn't done that earlier. Those jackets were looking really worn these days—don't retail stores KNOW I need pink clothes in October??

I was so rushed that I was almost late for my 10 a.m. radio interview at Cox Radio 104 with Daniel Baron. He was promoting '30 for Ana,' a 30 mile run that benefited The Rose. This was the third year of the event, something he and his family had organized to honor his sister, Ana, who had lost her battle.

I love being around Daniel. He's one of those good people who does things for all the right reasons. As we settled into our seats behind the microphones, Suzi Hanks, 104's best personality, eased us into the interview.

"Ana was such an inspiration," Daniel explained. "She was diagnosed when she was thirty years old and we run to honor her memory. We also want to raise awareness for IBC and funds for The Rose. We start the run at MD Anderson, go by the hospice where she spent her last days, and then head to The Rose. They have people waiting for us and we take pictures. It was The Rose who diagnosed Ana and got her into treatment. She had been misdiagnosed for months. She had a baby and the doctor she went to said it was just mastitis—a common condition after pregnancy. But hers was inflammatory breast cancer. When it didn't go away, she went to another doctor, who sent her to The Rose."

He glanced over at me, "If it hadn't been for The Rose, I don't know what she would have done, but they got her into treatment." He returned to explaining the event. "The runners leave The Rose and then head over to the cemetery, and that is where we have our closing ceremony. Last year, with only 25 runners, we raised $32,000. This year our goal is $50,000, with 50 runners."

When Suzi asked him to describe the closing ceremony, he turned toward me. "Dorothy has been with us at the cemetery every year, maybe she could describe it."

For the first time during the interview, I realized Daniel was having trouble. I could see his emotions hovering just below the surface, too many memories suddenly rushing in.

"Suzi," I said, "Daniel talks about running thirty miles like it was nothing, but that is one heck of a long way to run! The runners are exhausted and by the time they get to the cemetery they can barely stand up. But they are exhilarated at the same time. Last year, I watched them all run up to Ana's mother and father and everyone was hugging each other, then as a group they sort of hung onto each other and all knelt down in prayer." My voice caught. I cleared my throat and went on. "Last year Ana's son, Maverick, ran," I glanced at Daniel, "how many miles?"

"Twelve," he answered.

"Here was this little tyke of a guy, what is he seven or eight now, running right alongside his uncles and his dad. He was so tired, his legs were wobbly. But when he reached the headstone of his mother's grave, he touched it and said, 'Hi Mom.'"

My voice cracked again but I pushed on. "Ana was the first

woman we diagnosed through our Young Women's Clinic. We started the clinic in 2005 for women who are under forty years old. We knew we needed the clinic, every year we diagnose forty to fifty young women, and many of them have aggressive cancers, just like Ana.

"Ana was such an ambassador. It didn't matter how bad she felt or if she was having chemotherapy, she always volunteered to go with us and share her story. When Ana lost her battle, I really took it hard. I told her husband Gerry how bad I felt. His words were such a comfort. 'Dorothy, The Rose gave her another five years. Briana, our daughter, was six years old and has so many memories of her mother. And even though Maverick may not really remember her, he will know her because of all the stories—so don't ever forget that The Rose gave our family that time.'"

Daniel told other stories about Ana. Tears shone in his eyes when he described her last days and how she hung on so she could personally meet the newest addition to the family, her niece. After welcoming 'Baby Ana,' she said, "Now I can go," and two days later took her last breath.

After the radio interview, I sandwiched in two other meetings, then rushed to get to the Channel 2 studios by 3 p.m. for our phone bank.

When I entered, Karen was giving instructions to the twenty people who had come to answer phones. They were all bilingual. It was a mixture of Rose staff, survivors, co-survivors, and volunteers. She was prepping them on how to answer the phone and making sure they knew that staff was there to answer the tough questions.

Everything had been set up in a huge cavernous room, with overhead wires looped low and huge spotlights beamed onto the long rows of tables lined with telephones. Two cameras were positioned in front, each boasting a teleprompter. The words rolled in front of us, the same ones being read by the news anchors in the main studio.

We would be featured during the 4, 5, and 6 p.m. news, with cutaways to the folks in action on the phone bank. After thanking everyone for giving up a Friday evening to be with us, I talked about what was about to happen.

"Remember, this isn't a telethon or the kind of program where people are calling in to donate. We're here to provide information. We may not have that many callers or we may be flooded with calls, but I guarantee you will take at least one call today that will mean someone makes that appointment for her mammogram! For that someone, you being here may save her life!"

The next three hours flew by, and some 200 calls came in. News anchors, Dominique Sachse and Bill Balleza, came by to encourage folks to call in, but the callers were the real stars of the evening. Most were asking about how to qualify for a free mammogram, some had found something and wanted to know if it hurt to have a mammogram, others were curious about self-exam.

I handled the live web-chat. The questions that rolled across my computer screen were scary and poignant.

> *I've found something in my breast and I had throat cancer five years ago. Don't have insurance and don't know where to go. I can't talk so how can I make an appointment with anyone.*

Another message read:

> *My mother was the caregiver for her grandmother and mother, who both died of breast cancer. She talks about their courage and always focuses on them. I want to tell her that she is the hero for spending so much of her life taking care of them.*

While typing out another answer, suddenly I heard someone call out, "This person wants to make a donation!"

Brahana took the call. "Yes, it's tax deductible. Yes, you can stay anonymous." Then in a loud voice, she said, "Our CEO is sitting right here, I think you need to talk to her."

The male voice on the line sounded normal, but what he was saying was anything but. "What I'm asking, Ma'am, is how much do you really need to reach your goal?" Before I could answer, he said, "I want to donate to you. I looked you up and I have a lot of money I want to give away."

I swallowed. "Sir, every year, we have to raise $3 million to take care of the uninsured…"

He interrupted, "But that is just getting by, isn't it? Three million?"

He was right; three million was just getting by.

"Yes, Sir, that's what we need for each year, but can you imagine how that would help, to have that money at the start of our year? It would be a great foundation to work from as we raise other funds."

"Like I told the other lady, I want to be anonymous," he said. "I'm a professional athlete and I want to make a donation. What I want to know is this: What would it really take for you to make your dreams come true? To reach your goals?"

I took a second. *My dreams? My goals?* There was a part of me that was pretty sure we were being strung along, knowing that if something sounds too good to be true it often is. But that part fought hard against the part of me that has always been blown away by the unexpected and extraordinary generosity of people. I had nothing to lose.

"Our two-year goal, that would push us toward becoming sustainable, is $9 million." I stood there, holding the phone, hearing the words echo into the receiver. *$9 million.*

"Then seven million to start would help?" he asked. "This money would go to The Rose. And it would go directly to women, not for something else. Is that right?"

I smiled, more wary and more hopeful than ever. "Absolutely, I can introduce you to the women who you would be helping." Then something made me ask, "Why do you want to help us?"

"My mother died of breast cancer," he said, "I was twenty years old and it was hard for her, for her kids, for me…"

An old familiar feeling washed over me. I insisted that he take my personal cell phone number. He didn't want it at first, but I said, "I don't want you calling us up and having to push a bunch of numbers to get through to me. I'm giving you my direct line and I'll be waiting on your call." I repeated my cell number several times.

The call ended. Everybody nearby had been listening and looked at me. I shrugged my shoulders, and said, "You never know." They all laughed and we all returned to answering calls.

By 7 p.m., the phones had finally stopped ringing. Everyone was ready to go home. As I started to thank everyone, one of the volunteers stood up. She looked to be in her mid-fifties, early sixties. Her face was strong and squared; she wore little makeup and her long hair fell almost to her waist.

"I want to tell everyone here that my life was saved by The Rose. I have gone to their mobile units for several years. I don't have insurance and they helped me each time. Last year, I needed an ultrasound, but it turned out okay. This year, they saw something in the other breast and that was two months ago. I had my surgery and because it was so small, I won't have to have chemotherapy." She turned to face me, "I want to tell you thank you for having the mobile units and for helping women like me."

Her words were so genuine, tears filled my eyes and I struggled to speak. Before I could say anything, another women stood up.

"When I had a lump, I didn't have insurance." This woman was tall and beautiful and easily could have been one of the models I saw at a recent luncheon. "I had gone to somewhere else and they told me I needed a biopsy. They said they would call a place that might help me. I was so afraid, but I'm a Christian and so I prayed. I was in the car, praying that God help me and send me a rose and at that moment, that very moment, Sally called me to set up an appointment."

I nodded, and said, "We know Saint Theresa of the little rose well."

"Yes!" she exclaimed, "St. Theresa! Who would believe that at the very moment I asked for help, the call came, from my angel, Sally."

She smiled at Sally, one of our patient navigators, who had come to volunteer. "That was three years ago and I've been through my treatment, I'm a survivor now!" she beamed.

From the back row, an older woman stood up. Her son and daughter and three grandchildren had come with her. She didn't drive these days, and besides, they wanted to help answer calls. She was still in treatment; the tell-tale scarf around her head confirmed it. She said, "This is my second time with breast cancer. The Rose helped me both times." Her Spanish was much better than her English, but we all understood.

For the merest moment, no one moved, everyone was quiet, a small space opened up in eternity.

Another October had begun. The next day, I walked in the Komen Race. I've only missed one since they began in 1991. The following week, a group of twenty employees, patients and volunteers would be on Deborah Duncan's "Great Day Houston" lively TV show and on Sunday my recently taped interview with Melanie Lawson, for her show "Crosswords," would air.

Throughout the entire month of October, every day was filled with interviews and presentations, and more women calling for help. A month filled with runs, rallies and fundraisers, all awash in a sea of pink. And in those same days, thousands of women all over the world were hearing those words: "You have breast cancer" for the first time.

Hundreds of women were led to The Rose for a mammogram or to get into treatment. And most of them found us through some kind of miracle—maybe they heard about us from a friend, or they saw us on TV, or came across our mobile unit out in their community.

At the end of the month, we held our second annual golf tournament at the exclusive Shadow Hawk Golf Course. It was a fitting end to Pink October, a picture perfect day choreographed by our board member, Jeanne. She pulled all the right people together. Many had never heard of The Rose, but before the day was out they would become our biggest fans.

The new mobile van literally sparkled in the sun, a spectacular splash of pink shining against the greens.

Kim was at the tournament, and later told me, "I almost got up to say a few words to the crowd. I have spent much time pondering the importance of this to me and 'Why now?' When I was diagnosed I really prayed that God would allow me to live long enough to see my children graduate and get married and eventually be a part of my grandchildren's lives. With each item I check off I feel a deeper appreciation for the blessing of life. So I wondered—what if I had not been diagnosed early enough, or even worse—not at all? What if I had missed these special moments in my children's lives? Yet there are women all around me that are living with cancer and will die because detection and treatment had not been an option for them. That is why I felt a call to action. A time to stand up and reach out to those women who also want to keep the gift of life and to see those very precious items on their bucket list fulfilled."

Another memory I treasure from that Pink October was an email from Nyla. It was in response to a thank you I had sent to the development staff for their work on the golf tournament. I congratulated them on its success and acknowledged the incredibly long day they had spent out on the course handling everything.

Nyla said:

Dorothy,

To be very honest, I was concerned about working late and leaving my kids behind last night. My mind was baffled with the thoughts of unlimited homework and a social studies test due today. As soon as I got home, Usman came running to me. He told me that he had very bad news to share and he was very upset. His classmate and best friend's mom had passed yesterday. Once again someone so close to him got hit by cancer. He asked me if it is okay to cry and I told him that it was absolutely okay to cry. So after he cried for a long time for his friend's loss, he said, "At least you and your friends are there for some other kid's mom."

My kid understands!

Thanks,

Nyla

There are so many children like Usman. Only eight years old, he has already seen people he loved battle cancer. His grandfather had died three months before and his aunt, Nyla's sister, was still battling it.

No, the seven-million-dollar-man never did appear. Imagine the thousands of women we could have served if he had. But Kim's gift was very real and it is already reaching hundreds of women. I know she responded to something deep in her soul and I thank God she acted on it. She, Nyla, and Usman are among the many reasons I keep on believing.

Chapter 34
Guardians

Not long ago, I was touring a new donor through the halls of The Rose, explaining to her how a Feng Shui expert had selected our colors and how everything from chairs to file cabinets to desks had been donated. I guided her through the patient care area, pointing out that every piece of imaging equipment was top notch, the latest technology, and all available equally to every woman, insured or uninsured. My pride was showing.

My spiel continued as we walked to the physicians' reading area and I introduced her to our medical staff, sharing how we'd grown to five radiologists. I was delighted to find Dixie in her office. Meeting her was a treat for any visitor. Seeing Dixie's office was another.

Her collection of zebras sang out in black and white from every corner of the room, even her chair was covered in zebra fabric. A huge pink wreath, a gift from a grieving husband, covered one wall. On the opposite wall was an equally huge painting of horses, another gift from a patient. A dozen slips of paper sporting positive affirmations, all awash with Dixie's precise handwriting, were taped to the reading station. The radio played Country Western music. An open jar of pickles with a fork in it sat to one side of her work area.

Our guest gobbled up the eccentricities of the room and was immediately taken in by Dixie's warm greeting. Yet, on this day, Dixie's normal exuberance was forced. She made the usual pleasantries, fussed over our guest, telling her how much we needed and adored our volunteers. Then she stopped mid-sentence and turned to me. "Where did you get these cards? The ones you gave me for my birthday?" she asked. She pointed to the three by five inch greeting card standing tent-like on her desk. The words 'Powerful Blessed Warrior' covered it in bold red lettering.

She continued before I could respond. "I love these cards. I have put them everywhere—at home, in my office, here. I keep them where

I can see them. I really need more of them, Dorothy." Her sense of urgency was unsettling. "I want to give them to all our patients."

"All?" I asked. Those cards were expensive. My mind raced forward, calculating costs.

"No, not all of our patients, but at least all of the women we diagnose. Like the two women I consulted with today. One has inflammatory, it covered half of her breast. She is so young..." her words faltered and those blue eyes were shining, she reached for a tissue. "Both were young. I need to give them one of these cards so they can remember who they are! No matter what they have to face, this is who they are!" She paused a second before announcing, "And our navigators, they need them, all the employees need them!"

She thrust the card toward me; her hand shook ever so slightly. I looked past it and saw that the thirty years of telling women they had cancer had etched deep lines into her beautiful face. Those lines told of all the times she had sat with a woman, held her hand and given hope, even when there was none.

She looked up at me. Memories filled the space between us. I reached out and hugged her; she felt so small in my arms.

"I'll see if I can find more of them, Dixie." My voice cracked.

"Good!" she exclaimed, slowly pulling away and regaining her composure. She flashed that famous smile at us, and with a, "I better get going before they fire me!" she left the room.

For the rest of the day, her words echoed through my mind. *Powerful Blessed Warriors. We must remember who we are.*

Remembering who we are as women and who we are called to be...to accept the invitation to envision a different world, to embrace the challenges, to pursue our biggest dreams, to believe, most of all to know that against all odds we are the force of change.

There was a time when the role of women was pretty much confined to three categories: the maiden; the mother; and the crone. All important roles, but I believe that another role has emerged—one that will impact our world for generations to come.

There have been other times in the history of the world when women held the kind of power that could influence the future of entire nations: the ancients of Crete; the women of the Exodus; Mary Magdalene; and the women who financed a movement, the Council of Grandmothers.

But never has there been a time when there were so many women with the education, the power, and the money willing to use their resources for change. Never have we had the ability or technology that allows us to communicate across the old lines, to reach out to other like-minded people and to create new solutions.

Regardless of age, women today hold the keys to tomorrow. Most of all, women in their fifties, sixties, seventies and beyond are at their peak, filled with energy and vitality, and so many have a burning desire to continue to impact the world around them. I'm amazed at the number of women who have decided they are more than a dress size, more than a label, more than any of the roles expected of women in the past.

These are the women who understand their influence and aren't afraid to use it. They are the decision makers in their personal lives and their businesses. They are intimately aware that their leadership impacts the wellbeing of their communities. They have the power and they care. They have the connections and they use them.

They are the guardians to our earth, of our culture, and for our future. They are the women who know that whatever we are doing now isn't enough.

Guardians. Fulfilling this role is quite a task, but the women I know are up to it.

We must remember who we are.

Epilogue
The Rose Today

On a cold sunny day in November, 2014, a car careened out of control in our parking lot, hopped over the hedges in front of our building, and crashed into the corner office.

After the smoke cleared and the car was pulled out from under the shambles of broken glass and shattered bricks, we discovered the wings of an angel lying in the seat of Amy's chair. The tiny wings were from a ceramic angel that had been sitting on the windowsill when the car hit the building. The force of impact catapulted it across the room, dropping its wings in Amy's chair before smashing against the wall. That chair ended up wedged under Amy's desk, the same chair that Amy had been sitting in only moments before.

Thankfully no one was hurt, the driver was shaken but okay and Amy had left her office for some strange reason. I won't soon forget that Friday. The thought that we could have lost Amy or that she could have been seriously injured haunted me for days.

In the blink of an eye, life can change: an accident leaves bodies broken; a feverish child rushed to the ER in the middle of the night; a diagnosis of breast cancer…we all know of those moments when our lives are altered forever.

Over the past three decades, I've shared many of those moments with the people who make up The Rose. Employees, volunteers and board members, donors, doctors, patients and vendors, media personalities, foundation grant officers and corporate CEOs, the list is endless and I wish I could introduce you to all of them. They have taught me much, surprised me often, and at the end of the day shown me what it means to love without reason, to care beyond one's own world.

The staff knows why The Rose exists; they have met the women we serve. They do the mammograms or navigate the patient or schedule the appointment and they hear the stories firsthand. Some have fought their own battle against cancer or watched a family member or friend struggle through it. I've seen our staff turn even the smallest of victories into celebrations and hold each other up during times of unbearable heartbreak.

Our cast of characters is endless and I could fill a dozen books with their stories. Diana was our second employee, a true Southern Belle who beat stage 4 breast cancer and lived a long life. Bubbly ever-the-optimist Johnnie came to us as a volunteer and announced that at age 65 we couldn't possibly expect her to learn the computer. Before long, she not only learned the computer but became the manager of one of the centers.

Our mammography technologists have been extraordinary. Regina, always a favorite among the patients, was the first to master both mammography and ultrasound. Our imaging supervisors, Patricia and Jeanne, keep the centers humming. Long-timers, Sharon, supervisor of the business office, and mammography tech, Rene, remember those early days and continue to cheer us on.

I couldn't begin to list all the physicians who walked with us. Dr. Atlas, who was our first referring physician, believing in us from the very beginning. Doctors Willis and Streusand kept our pathology on course for nearly three decades. Dr. Vogel at MD Anderson was the one we turned to when women needed treatment in those early days. Dr. Theriault and Dr. Sutton, who were champions and supporters. Dr. Milner, who bought us our first fax machine and was a top referring doctor. If room allowed, I would gladly include the other 4,000 referring physicians who have trusted us with their patients.

Then there are the volunteers, the people who give the only thing in life that can never be replaced: their time. Those precious souls who show up for committee meetings or who are willing to stuff envelopes or serve up shrimp or pray for us.

People like Helen. The same Helen who fell out of that first mobile van and who we couldn't trust with a computer because she managed to 'lose' our data base, not once but twice! (Thank goodness my oldest living friend, David Butler, restored it.) Helen has never missed a Shrimp Boil, and more than once she's purchased tee-shirts for employees as an appreciation gift. But the volunteer job she did best was being my Master Mind partner and opening her home to our meetings. Our group has gathered at least once a month, sometimes more often, since the early '90s.

Some folks would liken a Master Mind meeting to a prayer group. And it's true we hold up the names of people on our prayer list, asking for their healing or pending transition. But being part of a Master Mind group goes beyond prayer and requires that partners understand the power of belief.

We don't offer counsel to each other or give advice. The only requirement of a Master Mind partner is to affirm each other's request—no matter how crazy or seemingly unreachable—we all agree to 'see' it happening. We believe in the unexplainable.

We hold a place for The Rose at each meeting, calling her "Ms. Rose" so that I will have my own time for personal requests. Ms. Rose has asked for the right radiologist to show up, for the right employee to fill an open spot, for grants to be approved, for equipment. There has never been a summer in all these years when we didn't ask for the Shrimp Boil to make more money than the last one, and lo and behold it has!

Two other mainstays to our group are Marnie, who brought Healing Touch to The Rose, plus hypnotherapy that cured me from incessant hot flashes, and Margie, who brings a sense of wonder or new discovery to each meeting.

Helen has been the glue for this group throughout the years. Her unwavering belief that The Rose could always be more, serve more, do more, has stood firm. That faith has pulled me forward when I couldn't see the path ahead or given me a big push from behind when I was ready to quit.

Years ago, our group started 'clearing' The Rose. Every six months or so, we meet at the building. Helen brings her sage smudge sticks, Marnie carries our special bell, the one we ring whenever we receive major gifts, Margie brings a drum, and I usually carry water that has been blessed. We move through the building, silently or aloud requesting all sad and heavy energy be released and replaced by good and healing energy.

Pam once told me that one of the things I brought to The Rose and into her life was an introduction to the metaphysical world. "Like when you tell us about Mercury being in retrograde," she explained. "Not that we really believe that planets in the sky millions of miles away could impact anything."

Not believe? I thought. I couldn't imagine I still had a non-convert in our crowd!

While Pam might not totally accept Mercury being in retrograde, she understands that the emotions present in most any healthcare agency can actually be felt. Enter a church and you can feel the prayers and peace that cling to the walls, enter a jail and the walls are hot with anger and hostility. The same happens in healthcare facilities, especially breast centers. Having a mammogram can stir up a lot of anxiety. Worrying about having a terminal disease creates its own unique emotions. Over time all those different emotions permeate the halls, rooms, and entryways. A clearing—done with prayer and reverence—helps.

There were a lot of good things that happened every day at The Rose, good things that are sometimes weird or strange, others that border on the edge of magical.

But then, I don't remember a day in our life at The Rose when we didn't expect a miracle.

The members of our board of directors have their own reasons for giving so much. For Jeanne, it was her long-time friend Eileen (who she ultimately recruited to the board). For Eileen it is that personal knowing of what it means to have support when diagnosed. For Donna, it was the memory of Dixie at her mother's bedside as she took her last breath. Hearing Bob talk of a daughter who survived and a niece who didn't always grabs my heart, as does seeing the grief that clouds Myrleen's face whenever we speak of Vicky.

On the day Michelle finished her last chemotherapy treatment, she stayed awake half the night searching the web for a place to volunteer. At two in the morning, she found The Rose. During her treatment, she had discovered that not every woman received anti-nausea drugs—especially those who didn't have insurance—and she was outraged.

The two doctors on the board bring a medical perspective. Ted, who was one of the first to join our Physicians Network, provides radiation therapy treatment. Kendall is a reconstructive surgeon and refashions women's bodies after cancer. Both are intimate with caring for the uninsured.

I've never known why Jim has given so much of his time and counsel to The Rose, and Tom is much the same. Two men who stay in the background yet shower us with so much moral support and guidance. Our newer board members, Marcus, Loretta, Cherise and Robert, all have their own reasons and serve The Rose well.

Corkey continues to gift us with a catered Holiday lunch, but now he is feeding over 150 employees and volunteers, a far cry from the number he fed over a decade ago.

You've met the old-timers, employees who have chalked up decades of service: Amy, Pam, and Brahana as they held the heart of The Rose in their hands, and Bernice, who has made such a difference.

There are newer folks whom you haven't met: Shannon and Jessica, both new to the executive team, and our radiologist, Dr. Mahdieh Parizi, fellowship trained, exacting and full of energy, now leads the medical staff. They are all strong women who will carry The Rose into the future.

Then there's Kelley, my executive assistant, who keeps the wheels turning and me sane. Kelley brightens my day with the words from my favorite song that starts with "Zippity do da," while making sure I'm on time and prepared for every encounter. Every CEO knows what it means to have a Kelley in her life.

Dixie comes to The Rose a couple of days a week. She has never lost her caring for those less fortunate. While she still has her ranch and horses, she's become passionate about motorcycles, owns her own

Harley, and now her weekends are devoted to taking long rides with hubby Todd.

While we've had plenty of men on our team, and we couldn't have made it without them, the majority of our medical providers and staff have been women. Seldom has a day passed that someone wasn't PMSing, or in the early stages of pregnancy dealing with morning sickness, or fighting menopausal hot flashes, and yet, day after day, the work gets done.

We wear many hats within the organization, but we are always women first. We are mothers, sisters, grandmothers and daughters; caring women holding each other up in bad times; stubborn women refusing to budge from an opinion; strong women consoling a crying employee, caring for an aging parent or comforting a dying friend.

Every day I thank God for the brave people who do whatever it takes to keep The Rose on course and moving forward.

Over all these years, a lot has changed. Digital imaging now allows us to detect cancer earlier. Options for treatment are so much better than they used to be. In fact, by the time this book is published, there will undoubtedly be another new screening or diagnostic imaging test, another treatment, another discovery of a gene mutation—all focused around breast cancer—all geared towards increasing survival.

With a fleet of mobile units traveling through much of Southeast Texas, we now have the capacity to quickly respond to calls from businesses and school districts. And call they do. Companies know the value of on-site healthcare and The Rose's reputation tops all others.

Insured women are coming through our doors in droves—more than ever before—they know they'll receive the highest quality care found in the best imaging centers, but they also know that having their mammogram at The Rose means something more. I watch our staff smile every time another insurance card is handed over. My folks know every insured woman means we'll be able to serve more uninsured.

But still, it isn't enough.

Believe me, I am thankful that we live in a time when it's okay to talk about breast cancer and mammography. I'm grateful for the Octobers filled with an over-the-top frenzy promoting breast health awareness as pink adorns the malls, TV commercials, and NFL players on game day. Awareness is vital—every year another group of women comes of age and needs to start screening—they need to know about the importance of mammography.

But being aware isn't enough. Awareness without action will not change one single thing—it will not save even one life.

I struggle with the fact that so much of healthcare remains focused on awareness when what we need is the commitment of dollars to actually provide services— screenings and diagnostic work-ups, biopsies, and consults.

As Rose Kushner said, "All the education in the world doesn't mean squat if there is nowhere for a woman to go to have a mammogram." And she said those words over thirty years ago!

Today, there is a lot more awareness and a heck of a lot more money, yet too many women are still going without annual screenings and way too many are dying.

And we can't wait on Big Brother to fix things.

No matter what happens with healthcare reform and the Affordable Care Act, access to care will continue to be an issue. We have a very long way to go—years of political battles, states that don't expand Medicaid, federal mandates that aren't sufficient or just plain don't work—before every person has insurance, if indeed we ever get there. At the end of the day, having health insurance doesn't equate to being healthy.

In 2015, we were again fighting the United States Preventative Services Task Force's 'new' recommendations, which were the same as the ones they pushed in 2009. Of course they were the same; they used the same studies they analyzed in 2009! They do not recommend annual mammograms for women in their forties "unless they have unusual risk," and women in their fifties only need have a mammogram every other year.

None of the major groups agree, including the American Cancer Society, the Society of Breast Imaging, the American College of Obstetrics and Gynecology, the American College of Radiologists, the American Society of Clinical Oncology; the list goes on and on.

If these recommendations are adopted, thousands of women will lose insurance coverage for screening mammograms. Even more tragic is that the published analysis (Hendrick and Helvie) using the task force's 2009 methodology showed that if women aged 40-49 go unscreened, and those 50-74 are screened biennially, approximately 6,500 additional women each year in the US will die from breast cancer.

I feel like we've stepped back in time to the 1980s, when our greatest challenges were educating women about the importance of having annual mammograms and convincing folks in general that the uninsured were not derelicts living under the bridge. Ironically, these days the uninsured woman is just as likely to be the woman working in the next cubicle or the substitute school teacher or the newly licensed real estate agent.

Breast cancer is the leading cause of cancer-related deaths for women worldwide. In the US, a case of breast cancer is diagnosed every two minutes and a woman dies of breast cancer every thirteen minutes.

Screening mammography works, there has been a 30% decline in the mortality rate—30% fewer women are dying of breast cancer— since the early '90s. That's when mammography started being widely used and was first covered by insurance. No mystery on that one. Without insurance coverage, women won't have annual screenings. Without access to care, women die.

And access to care continues to be the key to survival. No matter what, there will still be uninsured or under-insured needing our help. There will still be communities that do not have mammography services.

Everyone deserves a place where they are treated with dignity—a safe place, a healing place—a place like The Rose.

While I was growing The Rose, and 'she' became the center of my world, others were growing families and had dreams and a personal life to occupy the center of their worlds.

The dailiness of this work and the constancy of having to find three or four million dollars ar after year exacts a high toll. The times of having to sell one's soul to appease another funder, the denials and the setbacks, the real loss of life when the disease wins…all these day in and day out occurrences wear away at one's being.

Sure, I'm proud of The Rose. It's a miracle she ever succeeded and unbelievable that over 500,000 women, rich or poor, young or old, have found care with us since 1986. I try to convince myself that we're doing our share, serving 40,000 annually. But, in my heart of hearts, I know it isn't enough.

Every emotion pales when I realize that no matter how many women we serve there will always be more in need. There are moments of deep sadness over the things we were not able to do and the women who didn't reach us in time.

Even so, I am profoundly touched and reminded that throughout all these years, God has been present, working in and out of our lives. I've seen thousands of miracles and been showered with hundreds of moments of grace. I've witnessed the life and death of others from a front row seat and been humbled to my core by the courage involved in this journey. I have no regrets about giving so much of my life to The Rose.

Whatever good The Rose has done over the years has come from the support of people who cared. Whether they were regular people, famous people, working people, retired people, rich, poor, and those in between; the one common denominator among all of our supporters is that they are people who give a damn.

They all reached bravely beyond the confines of their own world, their own reality, and into another person's world and another person's pain or fear. They stood boldly up from the crowd and said, "Let me help."

The Rose has been blessed by women and men who care— profoundly; people who know at the deepest level that *There, but for the grace of God, go I.*

We celebrate every donation because we understand that each gift represents someone's hard earned dollars. We are intimate with that term: "hard earned."

We are thankful and we are also resolute. Our work is far from over. The Rose must continue to be strong, to grow, to reach out, and to serve.

Come join us in creating the rest of our story and giving another woman the rest of her life.

Acknowledgements

I hate to think what would have happened to me if Patrick had not come into my life.

These days, every weekend I can get away, I'm at the GMILY ranch with him. People tease me about becoming such a country gal. Heck, I never even owned a pair of jeans and never allowed the staff to wear them except on special fundraising days. I was a city girl who loved the hustle and bustle, the theaters and restaurants, the concrete and steel, and I couldn't have cared less about being anywhere else.

That was before Peggy introduced me to country life. Patrick loved to go to visit Peggy's place; he was at home with the cows and the gravel country roads. It was during one of those trips to Central Texas that we found our own little piece of heaven.

Patrick, the man who guided me through the crowds of India, who gave me my engagement ring in Aphrodite's temple on the island of Cypress, who hiked me through the mountains of Canada, had once again shown me a whole new world. His encouragement and being on the ranch allowed me the space to write these stories.

There are so many others who helped bring this book to life.

Karen Campbell, The Rose's communications guru, who believed I actually had at least one book in me, and Alexa Moffitt, my spiritual advisor, who is convinced I have a few more to write. Many thanks to Irene Helsinger, who reserved the first copy by handing me a non-returnable $20 bill long before the chapters were formed. Woof to Caroline Casey for all counsel over the past decade.

Thank you my sister, Mavis Morris, for letting me tell her story. Blessings upon my Master Mind partners: Marnie Morrison, Margie Murphy, and especially Helen Perry, who saw this book in your hands.

I'm so grateful to every one of the peer readers who labored through the earlier editions. Thank you to all of my ALF Breakfast Buddies for their encouragement: Ann Barnes, Ange Finn, Emilee Whitehurst, Linda Flores Olson, Michele Malloy, Rebecca White, Vanessa Wodehouse and especially Rochelle Jacobson and Karen DuPont for their extra support. Special thanks to Suzanne Cotellesse who introduced me to Max Regan, my writing coach. For two years, Max kept me on task. Thank you to Diane Reina for her artistic works, to Lisa Birman for her editing, to Susan Fowler for her guidance and most of all to Kelley Reece for never letting me quit.

Finally, to The Rose, aka Ms. Rose, who survived against all odds. I will be forever grateful that she picked me.

About the Author

Dorothy Gibbons has been at the helm of The Rose since its beginning. As a co-founder, she has lived through every legal battle, every emotional up and down, every horrible economic situation, and kept the place running from choosing the wall paper to buying multi-million dollar machines to testifying before the legislature, to sharing final moments with a patient and friend.

Her collection of stories reminds us that every living thing has a narrative; every living person has a story – most never tell theirs. Her book is a small concise history of the amazing narratives that breast cancer has uncovered in the midst of its own epidemic.

Dorothy is a business woman, community leader, author, wife, mother, yoga instructor, and speaker. Her non-profit experience spans health care, education and women's issues. Her passions embrace the studies of women's roles in world religions, mythology and history. Currently, she is learning to be a rancher.

For more information about The Rose:
www.TheRose.org

For information about Dorothy:
www.dorothygibbons.com